WINNING
AFTER
LOSING

WINNING AFTER LOSING

Keep Off the Weight You've Lost —*Forever*

Stacey Halprin

Foreword by Dr. Jane Greer

WARNER WELLNESS

NEW YORK   BOSTON

The Langston Hughes quote on page 226 is reprinted by permission of Harold Ober Associates Incorporated.

Warner Wellness
Hachette Book Group USA
237 Park Avenue
New York, NY 10169

Visit our Web site at www.HachetteBookGroupUSA.com.
Warner Wellness is an imprint of Warner Books.
Printed in the United States of America
First Edition: May 2007

10 9 8 7 6 5 4 3 2 1

Warner Wellness is a trademark of Time Warner Inc. or an affiliated company. Used under license by Hachette Book Group USA, which is not affiliated with Time Warner Inc.

Library of Congress Cataloging-in-Publication Data

Halprin, Stacey.
Winning after losing : keep off the weight you've lost, forever / Stacey Halprin.—1st ed.
p. cm.
ISBN-13: 978-0-446-58039-7
ISBN-10: 0-446-58039-2
1. Weight loss—Psychological aspects.   I. Title.
RM222.2.H2244 2007
613.2'5—dc22
2006035172

This book is dedicated to:

The memory of my dad, Harold A. Halperin,
who together with my mother gave me my first birth,

and to

The memory of Dr. Mark I. Lidagoster,
who gave me my rebirth.

And to the very alive Faith Halperin—
who never said no to anything and
stood by me through all my recoveries from surgery.
I LOVE YOU!

Contents

Foreword ▌ *Dr. Jane Greer, Relationship
and Sex Therapist*   *xiii*

Introduction   *xvii*

STEP 1 Celebrate Your Success ▌ *Say Hello to
the New You*   *1*

STEP 2 Keep Winning! ▌ *Make Your Game Plan*   *32*

STEP 3 Turn Pain into Power ▌ *Use It to Lose It*   *83*

STEP 4 Appreciate Small Victories ▌ *The Little Things
Are Everything*   *125*

STEP 5 Stay in the Game ▌ *You Have to Play to Win* *155*

STEP 6 Win One Day at a Time ▌ *Start Fresh,
Finish Strong*   *193*

STEP 7 Feed Your Hopes and Dreams ▌ *Make Every
Day Count*   *226*

Afterword   *257*

Resources   *262*

Index   *279*

Acknowledgments

To my brother Mal Halperin, who welcomed me back into the family with open arms after I had shut him out so long, and to his beautiful family, my niece Hallie, my nephew Scott, and my sister-in-law Adrian, and to the rest of the family—Halperins, Posners, Priders, Levins, Haykins, Garai, and Smiths—for always loving me, no matter what shape I was in emotionally or physically. Grandma Goldie and Bertie, you are not here, but I thank you for the time I had with you!

To my old friends who help me to never forget where I came from and to the new friends who help me forget where I came from. Paradox—but oh so true! Jordan Stone, Gabrielle Woodworth, Wade Wilkinson, Jimmy James, John Salvatore, Marianne Morehead, Elaine Miller, Alan Chapman, Jackob Hofmann, Hugh Kepets, Teena and Lester Gamzon, the Hebranko family, Carla Bajek, Steve Brusca, Lori Jones, Linda Kamp, Roy Bryson, Philip Cornier, Steven Eliades, Kevin Coleman, Phil Kaabe, Christine Newell, Lynn Goldfarb, Shermans, Parentis, Liz Correri, and to my friends and staff at JASA Cooper Square.

Oprah Winfrey—for touching so many lives and making a difference; for touching my life and changing it forever.

Lisa Erspamer—I truly love you. Thank you for giving my story a life of its own and opening many doors for me.

The *Oprah* producers: Patrick Riley (my hero), Ann Lofgren, Stacy Strazis, Terry Goulder, Sam McQueen, April Terrien, and Bridget McDermott.

Shirley MacLaine, my mentor—thanks for going "out on a limb" to give an unknown a leading role in your film *The Dress Code.*

David Ciminello—for "loosely" basing the character of Angela on me and showing a fat woman with such courage!

My Teachers—George Koller, for introducing the concept of self-esteem to me. Grace Turkisher Riskin, who showed me how to shine and to have chutzpah! Jan and Judy Wilson, for teaching me about addiction.

My Doctors/Angels—Dr. Amy Ojerholm, for not laughing at me when I came to our first therapy session weighing 550 pounds and told you I was not there about my weight! You taught me how to learn to live with happiness and so many other things. You give a very loving therapy, which is just what I need. Thank you also for generously giving your time and professional guidance to the people who read this book.

Dr. Andrew Elkwood and Dr. Michael Rose—wonderful plastic surgeons who have continued what Dr. Mark I. Lidagoster, with his wife Lydia's blessing, started. How lucky I am to have doctors who are not only top-notch surgeons but also have compassion and great bedside manners. I love you guys! Dr. Elkwood, thank you also for sharing your expert advice about plastic surgery and insurance coverage in this book.

Dr. Jeanine Albu—for always giving me the very best of care. I admire your total dedication.

Dr. Alexander Swisteand and Dr. Glenn R. Jacobowitz for providing excellent care and always having my best interests at heart.

Dr. Mark Lowenberg, Dr. Gregg Lituchy, and Dr. Brian Kantor, thanks for giving me my winning smile!

Stanley Salomon, my accountant, for helping me sort out my financial past and finally put it behind me.

Jeff Gautier—makeup artist extraordinaire.

Elaine S. Revis—for the best advice I never took!

Natalie Kaire, my editor at Warner Books, for having the belief in me that I was ready to write a maintenance book and for having the understanding and compassion for eating addictions and overcoming them. You are a beautiful person!

Janis Vallely, my literary agent—thanks for showing me the ropes and being very patient and kind with me. You made me feel, from the very beginning, that all this was possible. You are truly one in a million.

Toni Robino, thank you for literally taking the words out of my mouth. Your professionalism and talent as a writer inspire me and your spirituality as a person motivates me to continue to change my life for the better. Thank you for coaching me to reach beyond my limits.

Dr. Jane Greer, Dr. Denise Ariahna Nadler, Doug Caporrino, and Dr. Bruce Hoffman, for generously contributing your professional expertise to me and to the readers of this book. I most certainly could have not done this without you!

Mundi Smith, for going above and beyond to transcribe the interview tapes!

Special thanks to Florence Tannen and all the members of the Winners' Circle who shared their personal stories, guidance, and tips.

Zone Chefs for delicious low-fat healthy meals left at my door each night.

Starbucks at Cooper Square for giving me a fun atmosphere in which to unwind—not to mention pick up guys! lol.

Kathy Kang and the girls at Spa Belles on Second Avenue, for pampering me.

Drum roll for saving the best for last (if this was my thank-you speech at the Oscars they would have dragged me off stage already): to Faith Halperin, my mommy, my friend, and a woman I admire more than anyone. I never got to see the look in Dad's eyes to witness this success, so your eyes became even more important to me. To see you so proud of me makes everything I went through worth it! Needless to say, I love you!

And last but not least, my very best friend Gertie (my toy Pomeranian), who has been teaching me to get ready to let a man in my life by showing me how to share my life and space. Thanks for teaching me to appreciate the little things, like when you smell the same tree every day with brand-new excitement. And to my best friend Gabi—thank you for handing me my best friend Gertie. You will always be her biological mommy. lol.

Foreword

Now that you've lost weight, you're probably eager to paint the town red, but you may not be ready just yet! If you're like most people, your celebration for winning your weight war was rudely interrupted by the realization that you could gain the weight back again and possibly even gain more. You know this isn't an irrational fear because the vast majority of people who lose weight *do* gain it back within a few years.

If being plagued by that fear isn't enough, you discover that the new you needs a whole new set of coping skills that you rarely or never had to use before. You're visible, truly present and accounted for, and that can lead to feeling vulnerable and unprepared. Emotionally, it's the equivalent of running for your life, so it's no wonder that so many people who have lost weight eventually put the extra weight back on. No matter how you've lost weight, unless you're psychologically prepared and you're in the right mind-set to keep it off, the unfortunate truth is that you likely won't be able to keep it off in the long term.

As a therapist, I've worked with many people who deal with ongoing weight struggles, and the vast majority of them just aren't equipped to keep the weight off once they've lost it. They're often blindsided and tackled by new emotional issues that arise once the weight no longer covers them up. More so, the diligence, self-control, and strict rules they used to lose weight become oppressive and wear thin during the maintenance phase. Once they reach their goal weight and are faced with day-to-day living, the newness of it and the nuances that go with it are confounding and very often overwhelming. So unwittingly they return to the coping mechanism that worked for them in the past, which is using food to soothe their emotional distress, compensate for other pleasures they are missing out on, and fill the void and emptiness that they don't understand.

The bottom line is that until they learn effective methods to cope with the tension and stress in their lives and reconcile the issues that trigger them to overeat or eat unhealthy foods, they are fighting an uphill battle. It's only when they truly believe that lasting weight loss has to do with their mind-set first and foremost that they are able to stay on track and maintain their ideal weight.

After years of struggling, Stacey Halprin was able to lose weight and keep it off by changing her mind-set and achieving emotional balance. For years, millions have admired her moving and inspirational story. This is the first time she is presenting the wisdom and advice that worked for her as a program that can enable you to achieve the results you want and maintain your ideal weight. *Winning After Losing* works because it cuts to the true cause of weight gain, focusing on an effective mind and body approach that provides the guidance and strategies you need to support your ongoing success. If you have been fighting this battle to no avail, this book will be the solution you need. The advice is invaluable, and the secrets and stories from Stacey and others who have won their own weight loss battles are sure to inspire you to refocus your efforts.

Winning After Losing is a seven-step journey to better health and fitness—mentally, emotionally, and physically. It addresses the issues that can stop you in your tracks and redirects you to make the changes and adjustments that will support your decision to fully participate in life. This isn't a program of self-denial; it's a program of self-fulfillment created by greater awareness, self-respect, and confidence. By accepting that you are in control and by staying in the driver's seat with both hands on the wheel, you can learn to make smart decisions, take the right turns, and keep moving forward in your life.

—Dr. Jane Greer

INTRODUCTION

In order to win, you must expect to win.

—Richard Bach
Illusions: The Adventures of a Reluctant Messiah

I gazed at my reflection in the bathroom mirror and I didn't recognize myself. All my life I'd heard the famous fat girl compliment: "You have such a pretty face." Now I had the full package, the whole nine yards. Finally, my body was one that women envied and men desired. I was thrilled! I was getting ready to pick up some friends in my new Fiat convertible that my dad bought me as a present for losing weight. I slicked back my long chestnut hair with a gel that gave it the wet look and gave myself a high ponytail. I put on my enormous eighteen-karat gold hoop earrings and a white halter top that showed off my tan. No bra for me; not with these perky boobs! I laid on the floor to slither into my size 6 jeans and sat on my bed to put on my high espadrille shoes and an ankle bracelet and toe ring to finish off the ensemble. I was picture perfect. As I walked to my car parked in our driveway I couldn't help noticing a group of guys across the street with their eyes bulged out staring at me. They couldn't take their eyes off of me. I got into the car, put the roof down, and put on some tunes. At every red light I got stares. Only now it was because I looked hot, not because I looked like an elephant. This was a fat woman's paradise. I felt so unreal that I was sure I would never be fat again. Why in God's name would I want to stuff my face again when I could look this good? Buying clothes is my new high and today I am going to buy my very first bikini.

"Stacey, time for dinner."

My mom's voice brought me back to reality. I looked down to see I had eaten all the frosting off the Entenmann's cake and almost polished off a pound of M&M's. I had frosting covering all my fingers and under my nails. I was a mess. I quickly tossed the cake box on top of my bed's black-and-white-checked canopy (the hiding place for my secret stash) and washed my face and hands.

I don't know how many times I played the starring role in that scenario, but I do know that every single time I did it, I believed that was the time I was truly going to stick with my diet and be thin for life. Throughout my life I went on so many diets I can't remember them all, and I lost weight with a lot of them, including Weight Watchers, Jenny Craig, NutriSystem, the grapefruit diet (now there's a program with variety!), and even the cabbage soup diet. But I always gained the weight back. The only thing I never tried was diet pills. When I was younger my parents made sure I didn't have them, and when I was old enough to make my own decision, it was no! As far as I know, not one single human being who took diet pills kept the weight off. Not one!

I was a normal-size little girl and began to get a little chubby when I started school. I was six years old in my earliest memory of bingeing and feeling shame. I didn't know the word for shame then, but I sure knew the feeling. My mom was in the hospital and a family friend brought me a beautiful doll dressed in a skirt that was made of dozens of wrapped candies. I sat on my bed and ate every last piece until the doll's skirt was gone. I instinctively knew this was wrong and felt like I had to hide her, so I quickly threw the naked doll under my bed. I stayed chubby until around the time I was twelve, and then I started gaining steadily all through junior high and high school. I weighed 170 in grade school and 250 by the time I was sixteen.

I left school without completing my senior year because by then I had gotten so big (437 pounds) that I couldn't fit in the student desks that had the chair and desktop connected and I was too embarrassed to have my own special desk and chair in each classroom. The day the rest of my class graduated and neighbors in caps and gowns were outside on their lawns taking pictures, my father was cutting the grass. I remember feeling horrible about how he must be feeling. He was an attorney and the first person in his family who went to college and his daughter wasn't even graduating from high school.

My parents wanted desperately to help me so they sent me to the best shrinks and the best weight loss programs in the country. I attended Overeaters Anonymous meetings, went to Weight Watchers summer camp, did behavior modification at the Van Italy Center at St. Luke's in Manhattan, had three stays at eating disorder hospitals in the South, and enrolled in Duke University's diet program twice, both times for about a year. I sought help from nutritionists, diet doctors, psychologists, psychiatrists, and even hypnotists. When I was twenty-four and weighed more than 500 pounds, a new procedure called the gastric balloon or bubble came out and my parents agreed to let me try it. The doctor inserted a tube in my throat and blew up a balloon in my stomach that was supposed to make me feel full. A lot of people lost weight with this method, but I never felt full. I just felt like I was a failure and was ashamed that in six months I didn't lose a single pound. Eventually there was a medical recall because the balloons were exploding inside people's stomachs and causing health problems. Still, even with all the failed attempts, deep in my heart I knew that one day—if my body held out long enough—I would lose weight and keep it off. But I had no idea what it would take for me to actually do it until the day it happened.

The day the World Trade Center towers fell I learned the secret that everyone around me already knew. I had become immobile. I was trapped in my downtown New York City apartment building because I lived so close to Ground Zero that the roads around my building were only open for emergency vehicles. In order to get food, water, or any necessities (unfortunately, a necessity to me was a candy bar) I would have had to walk one block. And walking an entire block was out of the question. I couldn't physically do it.

That day, at my peak weight of 550 pounds, I vowed that if the world made it through this disaster I would begin to take my life back. And that day, I knew—without a doubt—that I would actually do it.

Looking back, I can see that the years leading up to that fateful day were filled with the worst days of my life. Every morning, I awoke to the nightmare of what my life had become and wanted nothing more than to stay in bed and pretend that life was not passing me by just outside my window. Many days I never opened the curtains because I couldn't bear the contrast between the reality I had created and the life that I was missing out on. On the days that I *did* leave the safe cocoon of my apartment, I was insulted by strangers, laughed at, and even spit on. I know the word "fat" in five different languages and have probably heard it in more than a dozen. But most of the people I encountered simply acted like I was invisible. They looked right through me and avoided me like the plague. It was almost as if they thought obesity was contagious and they'd "catch it" if they talked to me or even made eye contact.

Thankfully, in the midst of all the pain and suffering, there was some happiness. I had wonderful friends and supportive family members who loved me and helped me whenever I needed it—often without me having to ask. Even in the worst of times, there was some fun and more laughter than would have made sense to most people considering the dire circumstances I was often in. And there was even some sense of accomplishment from appearing in several off-Broadway productions and real pride from starring in the film *The Dress Code* with Shirley MacLaine and Kathy Bates. And yet, on most days and in many ways, I felt like the person buried beneath all those protective pounds was slipping further into oblivion without me ever having a chance to meet her or dress her up and take her out. So when that person—the real me—discovered I was a prisoner trapped in my own body, I knew that I had to get my life back or die trying.

That's when I started to seriously consider having gastric bypass surgery and eventually decided to do it. By then, I'd had so many failed attempts that supposedly worked for everyone else that I made my mother promise that she wouldn't tell anyone what I was doing, not even family members. I thought it would be bad enough if it didn't work for me, and I couldn't bear the idea of people seeing me fail again. That was probably one of the hardest things I'd ever asked her to do, since our family didn't believe in keeping secrets, especially about something as serious as surgery. My mother has always been and still is my biggest supporter, and even though she was worried about me having the surgery, I think she was worried more about what might happen to me if I didn't have it. I'd already been diagnosed with a hernia, I had type II diabetes, high blood pressure, and high cholesterol, and it seemed like only a matter of time until my body completely gave out on me. After the surgery, my mother stayed with me and took care of me until I was able to take care of myself, and the day that she left, I decided to test if the surgery really worked. Since nothing else ever had, I was convinced that this wouldn't work either, so I ordered enough Chinese takeout food for a small party and ate it all myself. I'll spare you the gory details, except to say I could have done the special effects for the projectile vomiting scene in *The Exorcist*. I felt so sick I'd thought I'd die, but I was also stunned and excited. Finally, it seemed like something might actually work! I still think it's better for people to lose weight without the surgery if they can, but I'm grateful I had it because it gave me a second chance at life. I knew that a lot of people who have gastric bypass gain their weight back, so I was determined to change my mind-set and my lifestyle to maintain my weight and continue to lose more. As you know, having gastric bypass is not a quick fix—it's a jump-start that you have to work every single day to maintain. Now it's been five years since I had gastric bypass, and I've had to work every day to keep the weight off.

You really do have to change your mind to change your life and keep the weight you've lost off for good. Learning how to weigh consequences, being willing to be responsible for my choices, and learning how to face and handle my problems instead of denying them are the most important things I've ever done and the reason I've been able to keep the weight off this time. The biggest difference between who

I am today and who I used to be is the way I think, and just about every person who wins after losing by keeping the weight off says the same thing is true for them. That's why the seven-step program in this book works. This battle is won from the inside out and it begins by being 100 percent honest with yourself and as honest as you can be with everyone else. (Except when it comes to your age!)

When I admitted to the world as a guest on *Oprah* that I had eaten every pound that I weighed, many viewers didn't want to believe it. Oprah said, "Stacey is the very first person to admit that she is what she eats. No one ever said that before." People wrote to me insisting that I must have a thyroid problem to have gained that much weight. I think some of them wanted me to make them feel more comfortable about how I managed to get so fat. But I wasn't able to offer them the explanation of a medical condition. I was fat because I couldn't stop eating. I was also depressed, but there are plenty of people with depression who aren't obese, so I wouldn't allow myself to blame my depression for my size. At least not entirely.

Because I was well aware that I was responsible for my weight gain, if someone had told me that losing more than 350 pounds would be the easiest part of my transformation I would have said they were completely out of their mind. But as hard as it was, losing the weight really was the easiest part. As I lost weight, I gained freedom, and that's what kept me going. Almost daily I could do something that I hadn't been able to do in years—things that most people take for granted, like being able to bend over and tie my own shoes. The first time I got on a city bus, I put my quarters in the MetroCard slot instead of the coin slot and the driver looked at me like I was an alien from another planet. In a way I was. The pièce de résistance was when I could finally cross my legs. That was the day I felt like I entered into womanhood. I was on cloud nine all day. Every new experience, from being able to fasten my seat belt on an airplane (without having to ask for the "fat person extension belt") to having my very first slow dance (just a few years ago) to buying clothes off the rack (instead of waiting a month for the dressmaker to finish the clothes I ordered), was a thrill—and still is!

You've probably already learned that losing weight didn't make your other problems go away. In fact, it's just the opposite. When people put the food down, the problems—old and new—come up. So your life may be better, but it's probably not easier. The most challenging part of my rebirth has been taking the issues and pain that led to my overeating and turning them into fuel to improve my life and myself. One of my biggest hurdles has been getting over the anger at myself and the anger at the way others treated me—or ignored me—when I was heavier. The way I started to get over my anger with others was by finally realizing that I wasn't exactly putting out the welcome mat. The vibe I gave out was more like, "Don't you dare even think of looking at me, or else!" I put up a shield of armor and God help the people who tried to get around it! Letting anyone new get past that shield was almost impossible for me unless they happened to be a gay male with a great sense of humor and a lion's share of compassion. Now that I think about it, I probably scared off a lot of people who could have been friends. I had a real talent for rejecting other people before they had a chance to accept or reject me.

Even now, it takes a lot of energy, total dedication, inspiration, motivation, and support from a whole lot of people to resist old temptations. There are days when I have to humbly put my tail between my legs and ask for the help that other people are willing to give me. But as hard as it is sometimes, I never feel like it's not worth it. How can I put a price on my life, my future, or my dreams? How can you put one on yours?

Mission Possible

I don't know about you, but I'm tired of being a yo-yo dieter, tired of gaining it back and hiding because of the shame. Whether you've lost fifteen pounds, fifty pounds, or more, let's end this cycle once and for all! I decided to write this book because even though there are hundreds of books that tell people how to lose weight, I couldn't find a single one that explained how to keep the weight off. I couldn't believe it. Not one book! Not one infomercial selling a weight maintenance program. And all the commercials for weight loss products and programs had people proudly telling how much they lost, but nobody saying anything about how long they'd kept the weight off. When I started doing public appearances and giving talks to different organizations, it was obvious that there were a lot of people who were asking the same question as me: "How do I keep the weight off forever?"

It was that question that motivated me to write down exactly what I was doing and how I was doing it. It also made me want to learn even more about what works and what doesn't, so I started to talk to people who were experts in nutrition, fitness, and mental health. My mission is to share what I've learned so none of us have to be part of the horrible statistic we've heard our whole lives! Depending which source or research study you read, between 90 and 98 percent of people who lose weight gain it back within a year or two, and many of them gain back more than they lost.

The plan in this book is based on my own experience and complemented by the insights of experts in psychology, fitness, nutrition, and traditional and alternative medicine. Thanks to these willing and generous professionals, including my own therapist, Amy Ojerholm, PhD (who I call Amy), I've been able to put together a survival guide that works. I should warn you that much of what you are about to read is not about food and exercise. Of course, I've included important information on those topics, but most of the book is about developing and maintaining the mind-set you need to succeed, not only with your decision to stay healthy and fit, but also with every other goal that's important to you. Whatever issues, emotional pain, or insecurities stopped you from being thin in the past will stop you from accomplishing other things that are important to you unless you face them and deal with them. The pain doesn't disappear with the pounds! Not only that, but life is sure to hand you new challenges and problems to solve, and unless you learn how to handle those things without overeating, you can pretty much count on being part of the dismal statistic of people who fail to maintain their weight loss. The reason most people gain weight back and the reason others are able to keep it off comes down to one simple but profound truth. You are not what you eat. *You are what you think.*

The secret to winning after losing is in your mind. You've had the secret to success all along, now you just have to learn how to make it work for you. Think of it like Dorothy's ruby slippers in *The Wizard of Oz.* She had the power to do what she most wanted to do—to go home—within minutes of landing in Oz, she just didn't know she had it. And at the end of the movie when the Scarecrow asks Glinda the Good Witch why she didn't tell Dorothy that she always had the power she needed, Glinda says, "Because she wouldn't have believed me. She had to learn it for herself." I'm not asking you to believe everything you read in this book. I'm asking you to try it and find out for yourself that it's true and it works.

What You'll Gain from *Winning After Losing*

Winning After Losing is about something a lot more important than your weight. It's about your life. It's about learning how to accept and take care of yourself, discovering how much courage and power you have, and doing everything you can to make yourself and your life the best they can be.

The book is divided into seven steps, and each step gives you advice and action steps that are designed to help you to do what it takes to beat the statistical odds and prove to yourself that you are a winner! Whether you have already reached your goal weight or you'd like to lose more, taking the steps in this book will support your success. You will learn how to celebrate and say hello to the new you, how to turn your emotional pain into power, and how appreciating the small victories and simple joys in your life can keep you motivated. You'll also find out how to keep winning when your plan fails, how to win one day at a time, and how feeding your hopes and dreams can keep you on track, even when other forms of motivation have fallen by the wayside.

I put the steps in the order that made the most sense to me, and you should definitely do steps 1, 2, and 3 first and in that order. After that, feel free to complete the other steps in whatever order makes the most sense to you. Just make sure you take every step, because every one of them is important.

Throughout the book, you'll hear success stories, observations, and pearls of wisdom from other men and women who have lost weight and kept it off. I call this group of people the Winners' Circle. Most of the people in it have maintained their goal weight for at least three years, and many of them have kept the weight off for a decade or more and are still going strong!

The book includes tips on everything from food and

fitness to beauty and fashion. Why are there beauty and fashion tips in a weight maintenance book? I'm glad you asked! The answer is because they were and continue to be one of the keys to my success. Too many times I see people give up on their looks because they don't like their bodies. They cheat themselves out of looking good because they feel like they don't deserve it. Even at my heaviest, I took care of my skin and coordinated my outfits, makeup, and accessories because it gave me hope that there were better days ahead. Taking care of my appearance was the first baby step that led to my giant step.

Every chapter also has a top ten list on important observations that I've made over the years. Much like blind people who develop their other senses more fully, people who have been overweight have a way of seeing and experiencing the world in a way that others frequently miss. Most of us who have been heavy gag at the idea of the *perfect* ten, so I decided call my top ten lists the Imperfect Ten!

To follow through on each of the steps in this program most effectively, you will need to get a notebook or start a folder in your computer for the exercises and to chart your progress. Personally, even though I use my computer for just about everything now, I think the old-fashioned paper and pen method will work best for this purpose. You can use any notebook you like for your Winners' Circle Workbook, but an 8.5-by-11-inch three-ring binder works really well. You can keep everything organized by inserting a section divider for each of the book's seven steps. Using a binder also makes it easy to insert exercises or journal entries that you do when you don't have your workbook with you.

Meet the Experts

Okay, here's the deal. While I consider myself an expert on being fat, I am not an expert on all the psychological stuff that you need to know to maintain your goal weight. I'm also not a doctor, fitness coach, or nutritionist. So what I did was find the best people to help you get your life together and keep it together.

Primary experts in the book include:

▌ My therapist, Amy Ojerholm, PhD, a clinical psychologist in private practice in New York City. Her special areas of expertise include psychodynamic and cognitive-behavioral therapy for adults struggling with eating, weight, and body image issues. Dr. Ojerholm facilitates a monthly Weight Loss Surgery Support Group at St. Luke's–Roosevelt Hospital Center and also sees patients at the FEGS Manhattan Counseling Center. She is an all-around powerful woman.

▌ Dr. Jane Greer, a nationally known marriage and sex therapist in private practice for over twenty years. She wrote the weekly "Let's Talk About Sex" advice column for *Redbook* magazine online and is the author of four mainstream books. She's also a relationship expert and monthly columnist for *Happen* magazine/Match.com, and she is a sex expert for Liberator.com. She appears regularly on CNN, NBC, Fox News, and elsewhere. Dr. Greer is a member of the American Association of Marriage and Family Therapists and the American Association of Sexuality Educators, Counselors, and Therapists.

- Dr. Denise Ariahna Nadler, founder and CEO of Healing Integrations and a chiropractic physician, international speaker, and transformational life coach. She specializes in the mind-body-spirit connection and assists her clients to live their lives to the fullest by showing them how to remove inner blocks and align with their inner voice and the essence of their spirit. She has appeared on the same platform as Dr. Wayne Dyer, Dr. Bernie Siegel, T. Harv Eker, and Mark Victor Hansen.

- Doug Caporrino, biochemist, fitness expert, and nutritionist. Doug worked for Orion Pictures as a personal fitness consultant for John Travolta, La Toya Jackson, Eddie Murphy, and Sylvester Stallone. He is the health and fitness advisor for *Live with Regis and Kelly* and recently completed a fitness video with the Dallas Cowboys Cheerleaders.

- My surgeon, Andrew Elkwood, MD, a plastic and reconstructive surgeon at the Plastic Surgery Center in Shrewsbury, New Jersey. He is one of the few doctors who perform unique operations involving nerve rebuilding and complex reconstruction. Not only is he a top-notch surgeon, but he's also always willing to listen to my hopes and fears and do his absolute best for me.

- Bruce Hoffman, MB, CHB, a pioneer in the field of optimum health. As the medical director of the Hoffman Centre for Integrative Medicine in Calgary, Dr. Hoffman is leading the field of integrative medicine and the emerging field of spirituality and medicine in Canada. Dr. Hoffman is on the leading edge of health and wellness.

Let's get started!

STEP 1

Celebrate Your Success
Say Hello to the New You

*The real voyage of discovery consists not in seeking
new landscapes but in having new eyes.*
—Marcel Proust

I adjusted my red sweater so that it rested just off my shoulders and my thoughts drifted back to my old fantasy of being a size 6 that used to replay in my mind every time I was about to start a new diet. Cherished as the fantasy was, I am very happy being who I am today. No way a size 6—not even my feet are a 6—but I've lost enough weight that I can rest a small object in the little nook in my collarbone. Now as I check out my reflection in the mirror I can't help thinking about how much my life has changed.

When I slimmed down to a svelte 190 my world turned upside down. (Yes, I said slim. Let's face it, when you were 500-plus pounds for most of your life, 190 is bikini weight.) Whether you've lost fifteen pounds, fifty, or a hundred, now that you have lost weight, you are probably seeing yourself, other people, and the world in a different light. This stranger in a strange land sensation can totally take you by surprise and trigger a wide range of emotions. Any time you make a big change, you need time to adjust to the new you. For example, for the first year or so after I lost weight, whenever people offered to pick me up and give me a ride somewhere, I'd ask them if I could fit in their car. I wish I had photos of the looks on their faces! It was hilarious when I asked that question to people who never knew me when I was heavy because they were so bewildered by the question that they had no idea what to say. After a pregnant pause, they gave me answers that had nothing to do with my size. They'd say things like, "I have a sedan," or "There's only four of us going. There will plenty of room." Every now and again, I still catch myself having those kinds of concerns because I don't always remember what size I am now.

Even though I've kept my excess weight off for more than five years, I'm still afraid that I could gain it all back. When I look in the mirror, I can still see the woman who couldn't fit in an airplane seat. I can still feel her enormous shadow looming over me. She is a force to be reckoned with and she's always right behind me. If you have a fat shadow chasing you, you'll be glad to know that this chapter is the first step toward a brighter future. As I've said, the secret to winning is to work from the inside out, which is difficult for a "beauty maven"! But it's impossible to do it in reverse, and have it last.

Step 1 is about letting go of the old you and celebrating the new you. In this chapter you will look at the way your life is changing now that you've shed your weight, and begin learning how to set better boundaries and speak your truth, instead of swallowing it. You will also learn how to deal with stress and how to expand your focus from your body to a much bigger picture so you can have a love affair with the world.

The Old You and the New You

Ready? Okay, let's go. The first step in winning after losing is appreciating and celebrating the new you. Easier said than done, no? But you have to know who you were when you were heavier and who you are now. Are your hopes, dreams, and goals the same as they were the day you started to lose weight? Or have they changed? You need to go over this in your mind and really be clear about it. Life has a way of changing things when you least expect it. Having this awareness will give you a chance to set some new goals and applaud yourself for those you have already achieved.

Just about everyone who's lost weight knows that the number of pounds they've shed isn't as important or impressive as how long they've kept them off. So whether you've been maintaining for one day, ten years, or more, every day of success is worth celebrating! Every new thing you get to experience as a result of having a healthy, fit body is also worth celebrating, and so are the things you couldn't do when you were heavier that you're able to do again now. Whether that means being able to zip up your favorite jeans, walk up a flight of stairs without losing your breath, or fit more comfortably into an airplane seat, it's important to give yourself credit and appreciate your success. Members of the Winners' Circle shared the following list of things that they feel most proud of. See how many of these examples you can celebrate and make your own list in your Winners' Circle Workbook!

Winners' Circle Accomplishments

Petra—Self-control.

Paul—Attractive women smile at me instead of looking right through me.

Sherry—My health. I just had an excellent health report from my doctor.

Margaret—I look in the mirror and love the person I see there.

Joey—I felt sorry for the old me, but I didn't like him that much. I love who I am today.

Emily—I feel comfortable in my own skin. I am able to walk without losing my breath.

Stephanie—I'm proud that at the age of fifty-seven, I still get mistaken for being my daughter's sister rather than her mother. And unlike many of my friends who are my age, I have no serious health problems.

Jande—I realized I used to have no integrity with myself. Now I'm accountable to myself, and that feels really good.

Mark—I used to think that if I lost weight my life would have too many restrictions. It's unbelievable to me that I actually have so much more freedom. I'm proud that I made myself lose weight, even though I didn't know then how much fun being healthy and in shape would be.

Vicki—I feel proud that my body is healthy and that I am more fit and toned than ever before. From a purely cosmetic perspective, I also love the way I look in my clothes.

Yvonne—I like having a closet of size 4s and 6s. Best of all, I feel very confident in any social setting. I'm not embarrassed about taking pictures anymore and I feel confident in a bathing suit—in public!

Larry—I'm proud that all my friends are continually amazed by my ability to take it off and keep it off. I am healthier and feel better. My endurance and stamina are fabulous, and I don't need to keep buying larger clothes!

Karen—Even when everything else in my life spins out of control (as it is now!) I am able to maintain control over my body.

Dawn—I have been able to complete three half marathons, and I have so much more self-confidence than I used to.

Patrick—I look at exercise and maintaining my weight as a personal challenge and a constant process for me to keep striving and improving myself.

Florence—I love the way I look and feel, and even though life always presents challenges, I feel strong enough to face them and do what I need to do.

Acknowledge Your Support Team

In addition to celebrating yourself, this is the perfect time to appreciate and celebrate all the people who have helped you make it to this point. Make a list of everyone, from your partner to your friends, kids, coworkers, neighbors, relatives, and pets, who has played a part in your success. Thank each of them for their contribution to your personal growth and weight loss. In some cases you'll be thanking them for what they did and in other cases you'll be thanking them for what they didn't do. "Thank you for taking care of the kids so I could go to the gym." "Thank you for not bringing home potato chips or ice cream!" You'll probably find that many of the people who supported you while you were losing weight will also be willing to play a supportive role in your weight maintenance. The maintenance battle is rarely won alone, so welcome the people who love you to help you to keep winning. (In chapter 3, you'll have a chance to recruit your Winning Team.)

Aside from the people in your daily life, you might also want to participate in some online discussion groups or chat rooms for people who are losing or who have lost weight. Sometimes it's easier to share what you're thinking and how you're feeling with people who don't know you. There's something to be said for being anonymous!

Before and After

As a starting point to seeing the similarities and differences between the old and the new you, Dr. Jane Greer suggests that you answer the following questions to give you a snapshot image of who you were and who you are now. She says, "Relax and let whatever thoughts pop into your mind guide you to your answers. Usually the first thing that crosses your mind points you in the right direction."

The Old Me
I used to see myself as:
Most of all I wanted to be:
More than anything, I wanted to be able to:
Every day I hoped:
If I had one wish it would have been:
My favorite dream for my future was:

The New Me
Now I see myself as:
Most of all I want to be:
More than anything, I want to be able to:
Today I hope:
Now I wish:
My favorite dream for my future is:

Your own answers to those questions are the only ones that matter, but I'm sharing Marlene's answers to give you an example of how to do the exercise. Marlene has been in the Winners' Circle for three years.

The Old Me
I used to see myself as: shy and unsociable
Most of all I wanted to be: liked and accepted
More than anything, I wanted to be able to: feel good about myself
Every day I hoped: something would happen to give me the strength to lose weight
If I had one wish it would have been: to be thin
My favorite dream for my future was: going to my twenty-year class reunion as a size 6

The New Me
Now I see myself as: confident and friendly
Most of all I want to be: healthy, mentally and physically
More than anything, I want to be able to: reach the career goals I set for myself
Today I hope: I live long enough to do all the things I want to do
Now I wish: I could help everyone who is overweight to experience the freedom and natural high of being in good shape and in control
My favorite dream for my future is: to keep living every day as if it's my first and my last!

Shedding the Invisibility Cloak

I knew my invisibility cloak was gone when a cab driver dodged three lanes of traffic to pull over and pick me up. In the past, I would watch one empty cab after another drive right by as if I wasn't there. (Imagine, if you will, being invisible at 500 pounds. It's an oxymoron, like the term "jumbo shrimp"!) The differences in the way people treated me once I lost weight were probably gradual changes, but I remember feeling like it happened overnight. One day people avoided making eye contact with me and the next day they were smiling at me and starting conversations for no apparent reason. One day when I was walking down a street in Manhattan by myself, a good-looking guy bought flowers from a street vendor and gave them to me along with a compliment and his phone number. That blew my mind.

Both the men and the women in the Winners' Circle know how dramatic it can be to go from being invisible to getting noticed, and not only by strangers and acquaintances, but also by family and friends. Even though they agree that most of the new attention is positive, some of them struggle with it because it makes them feel more vulnerable and exposed. Others have faced new challenges because their partners feel threatened by their new level of attractiveness, or the jealously of siblings and friends has driven a wedge into what used to be close relationships. Former "eating buddies" feel rejected by their thinner friends' new way of life and sometimes try to deliver them back into the jaws of temptation by showing up with cakes, pies, and junk food. We'll cover the emotional aspects of dating and navigating close relationships without your invisibility cloak in chapter 3, but for now, I think you'll appreciate hearing a little about what your peers and mentors in the Winners' Circle have experienced.

Mark said, "When women started checking me out, at first I would turn around to see who they were looking at, or I'd discreetly check my zipper because I thought maybe my fly was open. Seriously. I'm not kidding. I did that for a few months. I was fat for the first thirty years of my life, so when women started smiling at me and sometimes even flirting, I had no idea what to do. I felt like a schoolboy all over again, and not in a good way!"

Joshua, who had been married for ten years, said his wife Sheila had a very hard time with his new visibility. "I was in shape when we got married, but after years of having a desk job and hardly ever working out, I gained about twenty-five pounds. After I lost weight, Sheila noticed that other women—attractive women—were checking me out. A couple of times when we were in nightclubs, other women hit on me right in front of her. But instead of being mad at them, she took it out on me, like I was somehow asking for the attention and advances. Sheila is gorgeous and has no reason to be jealous of anyone, but for the first year after I lost weight, I think she sort of wished I'd put it back on. She's settled down now, but she still doesn't like it when other women look at me with open admiration."

Some of the married women said they felt very uncomfortable making eye contact with men when they first lost weight because they didn't want to be tempted by the attention from attractive men and they didn't want to lead them on. Paula said, "I was worried that after I lost weight I'd have to deal with men's advances, but not one man came knocking on my door! Sometimes I could see men checking me out, but none of them ever came up and talked to me or asked me out. It was funny in a way because that was one of the things I worried most about before I lost weight, and since it never happened, I worried about it for nothing." Karen, a happily married woman in the Winners' Circle, said she wasn't concerned because she knew that whatever happened, she wouldn't stray from her marriage, so she was able to relax and enjoy the compliments. She said, "More men hit on me now and it's the more attractive men, not the slobs who think that because a woman is fat she'll be honored to be honked at or whistled at by anyone."

Kathy, who has been married for fourteen years, said, "For the past five years, when I was at my heaviest, my husband had every excuse for not making love with me. When he started paying attention to me again, and making moves to get me back into bed with him, I felt happy and pissed off at the same time. It was really confusing. I mean, there I was the same person I'd always been, but when I was forty pounds heavier, he could hardly look into my eyes or kiss me. It took a few months of couples' therapy to get us back on track and to help me get over my feelings of anger and rejection. It was worth every hour and dollar we put into it. All I can say is that staying stuck in your anger isn't any better than staying stuck in your fat. Find a way to get over it and get on with what's most important to you. Now when my husband checks me out or when he gives me a whistle or a wink, I love it and I don't hesitate to make the most of the moment."

Most of the single women ate up the new attention they got from men, but some of them said it scared them because it made them want to pursue every opportunity and some were worried that they'd throw all caution to the wind and take chances they knew they shouldn't take. Kim said, "The first few times that handsome men hit on me, I wanted to strip my clothes off right then and there. The reaction was so intense that it sort of freaked me out. I won't go into details, but I will say that I did some really stupid and careless things in those first few months! One of my close girlfriends said I was acting like I was a teenager again and she didn't mean it as a compliment. One of my older brothers told me I was dressing like a hooker. That pissed me off so much that I wouldn't talk to him for a few days. But eventually the comments from people I trusted started adding up, and I had to admit I was out of control. I'm just lucky that I finally got ahold of myself before anything really bad happened."

Gina said she lost two of her best friends along with the extra pounds. She said, "One of them was heavy and we used to pig out together and she's still into that, so I can sort of understand why she doesn't want to go out with me anymore and sit there eating a whole pizza herself while I have a salad and a diet Coke. It still bothers me, though, because I never judged her or said she should lose weight. Just because I don't want to eat like that anymore doesn't mean that I'm putting her down for doing it. I have no idea what happened with my other good friend. She's always been thinner and prettier than me, even now, so it can't be jealousy. We used to hang out, go to movies together, and talk on the phone for hours sometimes. Now whenever I call her she always says she's busy and has this or that she has to do and she says she'll call me soon, but she never does."

Don't Swallow It, Say It

A very important part of succeeding in your goal to maintain your weight loss is learning how to speak up and say what you're thinking and feeling. Most of the people I know who struggle with their weight also have trouble being assertive and saying what they want to other people. It's almost as if they don't think they deserve to have opinions, or that they don't have a right to say what they think. This seems to go hand in hand with having low self-esteem and being people pleasers. They want so much for other people to accept them and like them that they're afraid to say anything that might upset someone else, no matter how many things these other people might say that upset them. Learning to appreciate yourself more, including your opinions, and being willing to set better boundaries with other people are important steps toward feeling good about yourself and creating the mind-set you need to maintain your weight loss.

Margaret, who has been in the Winners' Circle for several years, says, "I used to play this whole tape in my head that people didn't like me and wouldn't accept me. I didn't think anyone cared about my opinions or what was important to me. I wouldn't even give them a chance to reject me; I'd do it for them. Now I go into social situations feeling more confident in myself. Whether people like me or agree with me doesn't matter to me as much as it did before—even if I get a brush-off. Before, it would have crushed me. Now, I can get past it."

My therapist, Amy Ojerholm, says, "Learning to find and use your authentic voice is an important part of mental health and can support your goal to maintain a healthy weight." Here are some helpful ideas for finding your own voice and speaking your truth to others in a way that they will be able to hear what you're saying. Learning these skills will add a few more coping mechanisms to your repertoire, both in dealing with people you already know and when you are confronted by new people and situations that you are not yet comfortable with. These skills will also help you to communicate more effectively and assist you in setting healthy boundaries.

On Paper

One activity that is really healthy for everybody is writing in a journal. Amy explains, "Journaling offers a variety of benefits, but one of the most important is that by writing down your thoughts and feelings you are giving yourself credit as being a valid audience. Many people think, 'Why write in a journal? I'm the only one who's ever going to read it. Who cares what I have to say?' But the act of writing and reading what you've written can be very healing, especially if you're someone who struggles to identify what you're feeling or why you're feeling it. Journal writing is a great tool in learning to better understand your emotions and define what you're struggling with and what's bothering you."

She says, "Journaling can also be a very helpful delay strategy if you feel tempted to overeat or to eat something that you know isn't a good choice. This is particularly true if you have a sense that you're not physically hungry, but are emotionally hungry, and don't know what to do. If you can delay your snack by writing in your journal for ten minutes before you go to the refrigerator or cabinet, you give yourself the opportunity to address the emotional state that you might not be in touch with and there's a good chance that you'll decide you don't want that snack after all. Putting your thoughts and emotions down on paper can also give you a fresh perspective in figuring out what might be upsetting you or causing you to feel guilty, afraid, or stressed out. It also serves as a record of how you're changing and the progress that you're making. If you're stuck in a rut, it's a really good way to identify what's going on, how you're feeling about it, and what you want to change. Lots of my patients tell me how rewarding it is to look back through their journals and see that they have accomplished many of the things they set out to do—both big and small."

Journaling is also a great way to validate yourself. The support and understanding that you got when you were losing weight can quickly disappear after you reach your goal weight because people think the struggle is over. So you have to be willing to ask for what you need and you have to be able to take care of some of your own need to be validated. The unfortunate truth is that if you don't believe you deserve validation and are unwilling to validate yourself, it's much harder to get it from other people.

Out Loud

Amy explains, "When you lose weight, it's common for other people in your life to have feelings of envy that make it difficult for them to listen to you talk about your ongoing struggles. Not only is it sometimes hard for them to hear your issues, but it also makes them say things in response to you that may be unsupportive or even offensive. If you're talking to people who aren't getting your issues, it's important to resist the idea that your issues are invalid so you don't give up trying to communicate. What you need to do is find one person who understands you and talk with him or her about your struggles and about the others who don't understand you." If you can't find someone who really understands you in your circle of family and friends, I hope you will go to a therapist or join a support group. If there's no one you can openly talk to who can understand your struggles, it makes your challenges that much more difficult.

It's like trying to climb a mountain for the first time without a guide.

Whenever you make big changes in your life or go through a significant transformation, it's natural to leave some of your past behind, including some of your old relationships. If someone is pulling you down, you owe it to yourself to cut those strings. On the other hand, if there are old friends or family members whom you don't really click with anymore, but you still love them and want to keep them in your lives, there are things you can do to protect yourself from their negative influences and still maintain or even help the relationship grow in a different direction. (In chapter 3, you'll learn how to introduce your significant other, friends, and family to the new you.)

Meanwhile, a therapist or support group can help you figure out what you're feeling and how to deal with the people in your life who don't understand what you're going through. Amy says, "They can help you to articulate what your issues are and help you figure out whether you're doing a great job of communicating and the other people are just unable to be supportive or whether you're communicating in a way that's difficult for others to hear. There are many levels of communication skills, so it might be that you have a deficit in your communication skill set, or it might be that the listeners have a deficit."

Most people who lose weight get a lot of unsolicited feedback—both positive and negative. So it's important to learn how to state your position clearly and in a way that protects your own boundaries. At first you might feel like you're being rude when you ask people not to give you advice you didn't ask for, but learning to assert yourself in this way can make all the difference. Most of the time people think they're being helpful, and you have every right to let them know if they're not.

Here are some examples of unsolicited advice that might sound familiar:

"I know you like diet soda, but you'd probably feel a lot better if you drank more water instead."

"Now that you've lost weight, you could really show off your figure better if you wore different types of clothes. I'd be happy to go shopping with you."

You can establish safe boundaries by saying something like, "I appreciate that you want to help me, but I'm not open to feedback about that," or "I would rather not talk about that." If you don't feel like you deserve your own privacy and personal space, you can end up feeling very vulnerable. Feeling vulnerable can make you feel out of control and less able to stand up for yourself instead of feeling good about who you are and what you've accomplished.

Stop Stress Before It Leads to Weight Gain

An important part of getting to know the new you is learning how to check in with yourself so you are always in touch with how you're feeling. The old you may have reached for food when you were stressed, without even realizing you were anxious or overwhelmed, not hungry. For your choices to support your new goal to have a healthier lifestyle, you'll need to do everything you can to avoid slipping into "automatic pilot." In other words, make sure you keep your hands on the steering wheel and your eyes on the road so that you are present with each situation. When you notice that your stress level is starting to affect your decisions, be proactive and reduce your stress before it leads to overeating or poor food choices.

When you're under a lot of stress, you are not only more likely to overeat, but you are also more likely to eat foods that are high in sugar and fat. That's just one reason that so many people gain after losing, instead of winning! But you can stop that from happening, especially if you understand why it happens and how to combat the stress in healthy ways. Knowledge is power! Dr. Hoffman says, "Researchers at the University of California–San Francisco have shown a link between chronic stress and obesity. People who have a high stress level produce higher levels of the hormone called cortisol, which often leads to increased eating of high-caloric foods and sweets. When you have high levels of cortisol circulating in your bloodstream this will increase the mobilization of protein breakdown from muscle. Also, if the raised blood sugar is not used immediately for energy use, it will be stored as abdominal fat. This is why chronic sustained stress leads to muscle loss as well as fat deposition. Loss of muscle mass is a serious problem, as muscle is metabolically very active and thus helps to increase metabolism, essential for weight loss. As cortisol is increased it continues to raise blood sugar and lead to the increase of its opposing hormone—insulin. Insulin is meant to lower the glucose when-

HOT TIP
Don't Look at the Menu!

When you go out to eat, resist the temptation to look at the menu. Menus are like foreplay. They tease you and make you want more. The pictures are as enticing as the sexiest centerfold could ever be, and once you see them, it's almost impossible to pass them up. Decide what you will eat before you get to the restaurant. Some restaurants have their menus online, so one option is to check it out during the day when you're not hungry and make a decision then.

Even if you don't know exactly what a restaurant offers, you've probably eaten out enough in your life to have a pretty good idea what types of food different types of restaurants serve. For instance, if I'm at a diner, I know I can order an egg-white omelet. If I'm at a steak house, I'll ask the server if they have a veggie burger or a steak salad. When you're with other people, order first so you're not tempted to get what someone else is having. Be the leader. Remind yourself that nothing tastes as good as looking great and feeling on top of the world.

ever it is too high. If insulin production remains increased for sustained periods this can lead to a condition known as metabolic syndrome, a prediabetic condition."

He said, "An article in *New Scientist* reported that Kent Berridge of the University of Michigan–Ann Arbor showed that stress might trigger binge eating by changing how you value a reward. The study showed that stress might increase your desire for a pleasurable experience while not actually increasing your sense of enjoyment. In a series of experiments, they showed that stress magnified rats' desire to eat sugar, especially when the rats had a cue or tone to advertise the reward. It is a bit like seeing an advertisement for ice cream, which makes you desire it, he says. If you are not stressed, you can resist, but together the stress and the ad make it irresistible. Cortisol also interferes with a protein known as tyrosine, which is essential for thyroid hormone production. Excess cortisol leads to decreased thyroid function and a lowered metabolic rate, another problem in weight gain. On an average day, most people experience eight to ten major triggers to their stress response. Each time your stress response is activated and your cortisol level goes up you can experience an urge to eat something soothing or stimulating. Your stress response, also known as the fight-or-flight response, can be triggered by many everyday occurrences such as an upsetting conversation or interaction, being cut off in traffic, realizing that you left an important document at home, or not being able to find your keys.

"Not only can stress make unhealthy foods more tempting, but it can also impair your body's process of absorbing nutrients and digesting your food. Basically, the best time to eat is when you are feeling safe and relaxed because that's when your body can process and digest food the most efficiently and enhance your metabolism, which leads to fat loss."

Action Plan for Stress-Free Eating

Do:

▌ Eat while sitting down in a relaxed atmosphere.

▌ Eat at a comfortable pace; stay conscious of the process.

▌ Chew every bite many times before swallowing.

▌ Set your fork or spoon down on your plate between bites.

▌ Take a moment to feel grateful for the food and the person or people who prepared it for you.

▌ Pay attention to the internal signals that tell you when you are full.

▌ Eat in silence for one meal each week, savoring the flavor of each mouthful of food.

▌ Remember that food should be valued for its nutritional traits. Continuing to eat after the point of satiety overloads the digestive system, resulting in a buildup of toxicity in your physiology. (It takes twenty minutes for your brain to know that your body is full, so wait at least that long before indulging in a second helping.)

▌ Learn to eat food from all six available taste groups—sweet, sour, salty, bitter, pungent, and astringent. Each different taste has a distinct yet subtle effect on your physiology.

▌ Eat a few pieces of freshly sliced ginger sprinkled with lemon juice fifteen minutes before a meal to kindle your taste for healthy food.

▌ Eat freshly prepared foods. Lightly cooked foods are preferable to overcooked foods.

▌ Sit quietly for a few minutes after finishing your meal. Focus your attention on the sensations in your body.

Don't:

▌ Watch TV, drive, or have upsetting conversations while eating.

▌ Eat out of boxes or bags. Put your food on a plate or in a bowl.

▌ Don't eat while highly emotional.

▌ Don't eat unless you feel hungry. Think of your capacity for food as an "appetite gauge"—where number 1 on the gauge means you are famished and 10 means you are completely full. Eat when your gauge is around number 2 or 3.

▌ Stop eating when you're satisfied, or when your gauge is around number 6 or 7.

▌ Reduce your consumption of ice-cold foods and beverages, because these can significantly reduce absorption of specific foods by diluting the acid produced by your stomach, essential for protein breakdown.

▋ Do not eat erratically due to high levels of stress and a busy life. This will lead to inefficient energy production, weight gain, and obesity.

Practice Lowering Your Stress

There are lots of different ways to lower your stress level. For me, a swimming pool or any body of water immediately calms me down. Taking a walk, meditating, or window shopping works for me too. For you it could be yoga, dance, hiking—the possibilities are endless. Dr. Hoffman encourages his patients to do the following breathing exercise, which comes from the practice of pranayama. The beauty of this exercise is you can do it anywhere, any time you feel like you need it (no assembly required!). He suggests that you use this technique when you're feeling anxious or upset and when you want to quiet your mind. This exercise can also help you to relax and fall asleep.

Nadi Shodhana*

1. Place an index finger on the outside of your nose to close off your right nostril and inhale through your left nostril.

*Nadi means "channel of circulation" and shodhana means "cleaning." Nadi shodhana is a technique to purify those channels through which energy and information flow.

2. Place an index finger on the outside your nose to close off your left nostril and exhale through your right nostril.
3. Repeat this process three times.
4. Repeat the process three more times, only now inhale through your left nostril and exhale through your right.

Have a Love Affair with the World

While you were losing weight, you probably got a lot of positive reinforcement from the scale, the reflection you saw in the mirror, the way your clothes fit, and from your family and friends. But after you've maintained your weight for a few months or longer, the initial excitement of reaching your goal can begin to fade away. (No more parades thrown in your honor.) This is a critical fork in the road (pun intended) where people either learn to turn inward and rely on themselves and their coping mechanisms, or they get discouraged and turn outward, back toward overeating and other unhealthy habits. We can't let this happen! This is when we truly find out if what we said was lip service or really "This time I'm doing it for me!"

Beth, one of the women in the Winners' Circle, said, "I couldn't believe how quickly the people around me took my weight loss for granted. I had gained and lost my entire life, so even though I'd only lost twenty pounds, the fact that I was keeping it off was a pretty big deal for me. But after a few months, even my family acted like I was never overweight in the first place. The compliments died out, the encouraging words dried up, and my life started to feel like nothing had changed. I had said that I lost the weight for myself that time, but when the positive feedback stopped, I realized that I was still looking for praise and acknowledgment from other people. And then I realized that I wasn't giving those things to myself and I'd better figure out how to do that and how to enjoy my new lease on life or I'd be back at the bagel bar in no time."

Beth sums up the same basic story that I've heard from many women and men who are trying to maintain their weight loss—same song, different chorus. It also points to a very important part of step 1. For you to completely appreciate and enjoy your new way of living, you have to take the party beyond your physical look and the number on the scale and begin to have a love affair with the world.

Dr. Jane Greer says, "Your love affair with the world begins by discovering what gives you the most healthy pleasure and making those things part of your life. Start to look at what you like doing and what makes you feel good (aside from food) and plan those perks into your schedule. Get out your calendar and plan a small treat for each day of the week and something really special for the weekends. And keep on going! Stay open to spontaneous opportunities to try different activities and hobbies, meet new people, and learn or experience new things. This is an aspect of life where you can have as much as you want. The sky is the limit."

She explains, "The key to success is to feed your heart and soul, instead of your stomach. Think about what excites you and makes you feel happy and energized. It doesn't have to be something big. Remember, it used to be something as small as a cookie or a piece of candy. Feeding your heart and soul is about taking in nourishing emotional energy, and that means giving it to yourself and getting it from other people."

Dr. Greer suggests that you make a list of all the things you enjoy that have been getting lost in the shuffle and make them priorities. Just like you plan healthy meals instead of grabbing snacks on the run, it's important to put time and energy into the people and activities that are most meaningful to you and help you to feel good about yourself. For example, if you've been wanting to take a relaxing bath, spend an hour with a friend, get a massage, have a manicure, or just take some quiet time to read or watch your favorite TV show, *schedule it for a specific day and time.* Write it down in your day planner or Palm Pilot and keep the appointments as you keep appointments with your coworkers, doctor, or your hair salon. She says, "Many times people feel guilty about taking care of themselves and let everyone and everything else come before them. The trouble is that if you do this you end up feeling depleted and deprived and both of those feelings can trigger a desire to fill your emotional needs with food."

If you like reading magazines, but your stack of magazines is piling up and collecting dust, start with the one on top, tear out the articles you want to read, and carry them in your handbag, briefcase, or car. When you're in line at the store, waiting to pick up your kids, sitting in a doctor's office, or waiting for a meeting to start, pull out one of the articles and read it. By doing these sorts of things, you feed and nourish yourself in ways that go beyond food. And you feel a sense of accomplishment in knowing you are taking care of your own wants and desires.

Treat Yourself Like Royalty

A wonderful way to celebrate the new you and reinforce your self-esteem and your self-worth is to treat yourself like

---

HOT TIP
Smile and the World Smiles with You!

For me, putting my best face forward means taking care of my teeth. They were in terrible shape from eating tons of sugar, so one of the first things I did after losing weight was find a dentist to repair and restore my smile. I also had my teeth whitened. (If you're thinking you can't afford to have proper dental care, I say you can't afford not to. Turn every stone until you find a way to get it done.) Now taking care of my teeth is one of my highest priorities. I brush and floss at least two times a day and I drink coffee with a straw so I don't stain my teeth. Certain shades of lipstick like coral and red will also show off the brilliance of your smile.

---

royalty. You've worked hard to get to this point and you deserve to reward yourself and feel like a queen or a king as often as you can. The better you treat yourself, the more you start to believe that you deserve to be treated well—and then the better you treat yourself. You've been caught in enough vicious cycles in your life to know how a cycle works. So use that know-how to create a victory cycle. Now that's beauty!

If you have a budget that will allow you to spend some money on your own pleasure and comforts, take advantage of it. If you don't, you can still treat yourself like you treat your best houseguests without spending a dime. Think of it as four-star living on a shoestring budget. Use the thick, fluffy towels you keep in the back of the closet for company. Eat dinner on your favorite plates. Use your china and crystal. Spend time in your living room when you don't have company. (There's a reason it's called a living room! Make the name fit.) Take the plastic covers off your furniture and find out how comfortable it is without them. Sit on your sofa, or better yet, lounge on it, instead of just admiring it when you walk by. Wear the clothing and perfume you're saving for a hot date or a special occasion and sleep in your sexiest nightgowns, even when you're alone. (You can't feel good in your sleep shirt that has food stains on it!) Recycle your jumbo plastic tumbler and drink from pretty glasses that you like to look at and hold. Pull your best handbags out of storage and wash your hands with those pretty little soaps that are collecting dust in your guest bathroom. Say good-bye to depriving yourself of life's finer things, beginning with the ones under your own roof, and say hello to celebrating the new you and your new way of life!

THE IMPERFECT TEN

The Top Ten Things That People in the Winners' Circle Have in Common

People who stick to a healthy game plan and keep the weight off have some important things in common. This list isn't based on scientific research or surveys, and it may cause some unwanted side effects, like rolling eyes, whining, and moaning.

In no official order:

1. They believe in every fiber of their being that they can keep the weight off. No matter how many times they've failed in the past, they know this time is different, even if they don't make that claim to others.
2. When they need help, they admit it and get it. They never fool themselves into believing they can go it alone.
3. They plan ahead and don't let themselves get into food situations that might make them give up control, and they stick to their plan. They don't care how many people roll their eyes when they order olive oil, no butter, or salad with the dressing on the side.

4. If they stray from their food plan, at the very next mealtime, they eat healthy. Even if they ate a row of Oreos, they get right back on track. They don't say, "I blew it so I might as well keep eating." They don't starve themselves after bingeing to make up for the calories, because the winners know it *does not work*. (Starving will eventually lead to tilting back the fridge!)

5. They weigh themselves, but not obsessively. (If you're asking, "How often is obsessive?" you're probably weighing yourself too much.)

6. They never shop for groceries or go to a party hungry. They are well aware that's an accident waiting to happen.

7. They practice forgiveness for themselves and for others. They know that harboring bad feelings will eventually lead to harboring unwanted pounds.

8. They have a strong reason for wanting to maintain their healthy weight.

9. They practice living in the moment. They don't allow themselves to dwell on the past or the future.

10. They don't say, "Sure, Oprah can be thin because she can afford a personal trainer and a cook!" (No one burns the calories for her.)

STEP 2

··························

Keep Winning!
Make Your Game Plan

Once a man has made a commitment to a way of life,
he puts the greatest strength in the world behind him.
It's something we call heart power. Once a man has made
this commitment, nothing can stop him short of success.

—Vince Lombardi, former coach of the
Green Bay Packers

One reason people gain back the pounds they've shed is they don't create a winning plan to maintain their goal weight. If you're telling yourself that you can maintain your current weight but you don't know how you're going to do it, you probably have a case of wishful thinking. Spare yourself the agony of defeat by being brutally honest with yourself right here, right now. Unless you make an effective plan for keeping the weight off and stick with that plan, the only thing that will stay slim is your chance of maintaining your weight loss.

In the past, every time I lost weight I gained it back. I never had a maintenance plan. I just thought I had to starve myself. I didn't understand how important it is to exercise and I didn't know the right foods to eat or the right amounts. As soon as I started to feel upset, depressed, angry, or deprived, I'd order enough food for a dinner party and eat most of it myself. I had Chinese guys knocking on my door in the middle of the night trying to collect the money I owed their restaurants. I bounced checks at the local diners and pizza parlors and eventually I packed all the pounds back on, plus more of them. This last time I was able to keep it off only because I made a firm decision that I was willing to do whatever I had to do and learn whatever I had to learn to keep the weight off forever. I guarantee you that your mind-set will have the biggest effect on whether you keep the weight off or not. That's why the mental part of your plan is just as important as the food and fitness. Times can get very rough. Trust me that you must be prepared to have the best chance!

According to a study done by the Department of Psychiatry at the University of Pittsburgh Medical School, people regain weight, at least in part, because they don't stick with a maintenance plan. The great thing about those results is they show that people don't just mysteriously regain weight. It happens because they are not doing what they need to do to keep the weight off. That means that as long as you control what you do and don't do, you can make the right choices to keep the weight off forever.

But believe me when I tell you that there is no coasting in the maintenance game and there is no finish line. There is never a point where you can safely say, "Okay, I'm thin now so I can eat whatever I want and only exercise when I feel like it." Sorry, but it just doesn't work that way. If you sincerely want to keep the weight off, you have to make a plan that is structured enough and flexible enough that it will serve you for life.

The results of the same study also showed that people who keep the weight off for several years usually have a greater chance of keeping it off in the future. That is very good news! Many of the veterans in the Winners' Circle (those who have kept the weight off for more than five years) say that their new lifestyle, which includes nutritious low-fat food, plenty of physical fitness, and maintaining their mental health, is now second nature. Even though the first few years of maintaining their weight were in some ways more challenging than losing the weight, once their maintenance plan became a natural way of life, they were able to keep it up without having to constantly think about it. Personally, I can't wait to have a little more serenity in my life! Remember, though, that the people who keep winning don't let serenity turn into cockiness. They are forever vigilant!

The winners accept full responsibility for their choices and they stay in the driver's seat at all times—meaning that they don't even eat one doughnut by default. That doesn't mean they never eat a doughnut. It means that they control when they will eat a doughnut instead of letting the urge control them. It means they plan exercise into their lives instead of fitting it in when or if they can. And they are proving that with a solid game plan, commitment to that plan, and a strong support team, they can win the game! That's not to say you will never fall off the wagon and eat a doughnut mindlessly, but you will even have a plan for that and how to handle it.

Step 2 guides you through the process of designing a winning game plan that is tailor made for you! Your program should be as personal as your signature—no two exactly alike. You will learn how to plan to win by laying a groundwork for your maintenance plan that supports both your body and your mind. You will discover that you can make food and fitness your friends by making choices that help you feel your best. So you don't go overboard trying to make too many changes at once, you'll learn how to balance improvement with acceptance and how to have more control of your day and your mental health by writing your own script. You'll also learn how to make plans instead of excuses and get some real pearls of wisdom on beating the odds from the Winners' Circle. If someone has maintained her weight for years, believe me, I want to know everything she has to say!

Plan to Win

Believing that you can succeed is probably the most important part of any winning plan. Dr. Nadler says that one of the most frequently forgotten aspects of health and wellness is the mind-body connection. She says, "Through research and science we now know with certainty that there is a correlation between our thoughts and emotions and our body—a mind-body connection. The mind-body can best be viewed as one whole entity rather than considered separate and distinct parts. This point of view was put forward a century ago by William James, the father of American psychology, and has been affirmed time and time again by brain researchers, scientists, and doctors. (There are also many books that address the mind-body connection, such as *Molecules of Emotion* by Candace B. Pert, PhD.) What we now know is that how you think and what you think about, you tend to bring about." All the people I look up to in the entertainment field have seen and known about their successful futures long before we did. Hell, I knew I was writing a book at fifteen years old. You must be able to see what you want. There are still things I cannot envision, and those are the things I am working on the hardest now.

For most people, the mental part of this game is the most challenging, especially in the beginning. Your belief system, the way you think, what you read, the TV shows and movies you watch, and the people you spend time with can have a huge effect on your success or failure. Personally, I couldn't have made it this far without my shrink, the *Oprah* show, and Dr. Phil! Good old SUNY Oprah! That's the "college" I graduated from!

It's crucial to have plenty of ideas on hand and lots of activities planned ahead of time, so you won't be caught off guard and you can keep your mind in winning mode. In addition to including some of the stress-reducing practices that you learned in chapter 1, also plan activities that you love to do—things that make you smile, feel joyful, and just want to get up each day. That is one of the best ways to feel full of energy. Do you love to dance, sing, or play an instrument? Are there playful or silly things that you used to love but haven't done since you were a child, like splashing your feet in puddles, playing in the mud, catching snowflakes on your tongue, or making snow angels or sand castles? (I love making snow angels now that my angels are not fat angels, and just last summer I bought a huge jar of bubbles and went on my roof and blew my mind.)

When was the last time you laughed so hard that you couldn't stop? Laughter is a fantastic stress reducer and really is one of the best medicines. Definitely make laughter and comedy part of your game plan! How about music, books, TV shows, and movies that inspire you? Just like you plan your food and fitness, plan your frame of mind, because keeping your determination strong and staying motivated will make your plan easier to maintain and more successful. Remember, your mind determines whether or not to eat healthy foods, not your stomach.

A lot of self-improvement books offer one basic plan that is supposed to work for everyone. But anyone who's been fat knows that the notion of "one size fits all" is false advertising! There's no way that a generic maintenance plan will work as well for you as a plan that you create based on your own goals, strengths, and weaknesses.

Now is a good time to think about whether the weight you are right now is the best weight for you. Some people find that their goal weight is a little too low for them to comfortably maintain for a lifetime. If it's taking every ounce of your energy to maintain your weight, you might be better off going up a few pounds so the weight you choose to live at isn't such a constant struggle. If you feel that you'd like to lose more weight, consider maintaining the weight you are now for several months or even longer before losing more. That will give your body a chance to adjust and your mind some time to catch up with the changes that you've already made.

Game Plan Assessment

Take out your Winners' Circle Workbook and complete the following assessment.

Today's date is:

1. Today, I weigh:
2. My measurements are:
3. My clothing sizes are:
4. Note whether you are at your goal weight or whether you plan to lose more weight. (If you are planning to lose more weight, write down your goal weight.)
5. Explain how you will monitor your maintenance (or weight loss) to ensure that you are winning. (Some options include weighing yourself daily or weekly, checking your body measurements weekly or monthly, having your body mass index tested to monitor your muscle mass and your body fat, and trying on a particular outfit every few weeks to make sure it isn't getting any tighter. Your pants never lie!)

Make Food and Fitness Your Friends

To stay in the Winners' Circle, you have to figure out what foods are best for you and what types of exercise you enjoy. Discovering the answers to those two questions is like being handed the keys to the kingdom!

To find out the healthiest weight range for your height and body frame size, consult a few of the online sources, such as www.healthchecksystems.com or www.thecolumn.org.

Nutrition for Life

No matter what diet you used to lose weight, you probably need to modify it or possibly incorporate more variety into your food lists so you'll have a well-rounded nutrition plan that will support your long-term weight maintenance goals. Most yo-yo dieters know from past experience that it's tough to stay on a particular diet indefinitely, and making the transition from the diet to everyday maintenance can be very tricky. (If it was easy, we'd have lost weight once and never gained it back.) It will take time, patience, and practice to figure out the right amount of food to eat in order not to gain, but to maintain. But once you know the right amount—and you will—it will add great peace to your life! The suggestions in this chapter are standard, middle-of-the-road guidelines for healthy eating and are designed to give you enough flexibility so you can follow them forever. They are also helpful to review if you find that you've fallen off track with your eating habits.

The winning mind-set for food is eating to live, instead of living to eat. The people in the Winners' Circle consistently eat a low-fat diet. They also usually have the same healthy eating pattern on weekends that they have during the week. They cut themselves a little slack on holidays and special occasions, but they continually monitor the balance between the calories they eat and the calories they burn. Be very careful of becoming too rigid, because that could eventually set you up to fail.

The challenge with giving you information about food and nutrition is that expert advice varies far and wide, depending whom you listen to or which resource you go by. Nutritional needs are also different for "healthy" people than for people who are recovering from injuries or have illnesses or diseases as well as for people who have had gastric bypass surgery. If you're pregnant or nursing, your nutritional needs are different too. Even vitamins and supplements need to be individualized depending on your needs and also because they rely on each other to do the best job. For instance, your body won't be able to effectively use vitamin C unless you also get enough calcium. (Oranges have both!) These are all reasons to make learning more about nutrition part of your winning game plan. Knowledge is power, so learn all you need to know!

With that said, there are some basic nutrition guidelines that seem to hold up across the board. Use the following information as a starting point, keep track of what works best for you, and make adjustments when you need them.

According to the U.S. Department of Agriculture, a healthy diet:

- Emphasizes fruits, vegetables, whole grains, and fat-free or low-fat milk and milk products;
- Includes lean meats, poultry, fish, beans, eggs, and nuts; and
- Is low in saturated fats, trans fats, cholesterol, salt (sodium), and added sugars.

The Building Blocks of Nutrition

The four basic building blocks for optimum nutrition are water, carbohydrates, proteins, and fats.

Water

Your body is two-thirds water. People don't think of water as a nutrient, but it is necessary for every body function. You need water to be able to digest food, absorb nutrients, keep your blood circulating properly, and be able to use water-soluble vitamins. Water is essential for transporting nutrients into and through the body and exporting waste products. It is also needed for your body to maintain its proper temperature.

Carbohydrates

Carbohydrates provide your body with the energy it needs to function properly. They are divided into two groups—simple and complex. About 45 to 50 percent of your daily calories should come from carbohydrates and 10 percent of those or less should be from simple carbohydrates. These include fructose (sugar from fruit), sucrose (refined sugar), and lactose (milk sugar). Fruits are one of the best and healthiest choices of simple carbohydrates.

Complex carbohydrates include plant foods that have fiber and starch. Vegetables, whole grains, peas, and beans are all rich sources. By eating primarily complex carbohydrates you should be able to consume 25 grams of fiber each day, which is the daily minimum recommended by many nutritionists.

Your best sources of carbohydrates are unrefined fruits, vegetables, peas, beans, and whole-grain products. Opt for organic fresh produce when possible. When you can't get fresh fruits and vegetables, frozen or canned can be okay, but make sure they don't have added sugar, artificial sweeteners, or sauces. Whole grains, such as brown rice, oatmeal, millet, amaranth, and whole-grain breads are much better for you than refined grains such as processed cereals, white rice, and white bread. Refined foods, such as candy, soft drinks, sugar, and desserts, have few, if any, of the vitamins and minerals you need to get from eating carbohydrates.

Proteins

Protein is needed for growth, and it gives you energy and is essential for your body to manufacture antibodies, hormones, enzymes, and tissues. There are complete proteins and incomplete proteins. Complete proteins are found in meat, fish, poultry, soybean products such as tofu and soymilk, eggs, yogurt, cheese, and milk from cows or goats. Incomplete proteins are found in grains, legumes, nuts, seeds, and green leafy vegetables.

Some of the healthiest proteins are the result of combining partial-protein foods to make what is called complementary protein. Complementary protein gives you all the essential amino acids (the compounds that bond together to form protein) that you need. For example, beans or brown rice eaten separately do not make a complete protein, but if you eat them together, they do! Aside from brown rice, you can also combine beans with corn, nuts, seeds, or whole wheat to make a complete protein. Or you can eat brown rice with beans, nuts, seeds, or wheat to make a complete protein.

How much protein you need each day is no longer an easy question to answer because there are conflicting views. One thing that is for sure, though, is that most experts agree that we don't need to eat as much protein as people used to believe we needed. Not too long ago, the U.S. Recommended Daily Allowance (RDA) was over 100 grams per day. Now it is suggested that about 30 to 40 percent of your daily nutrition come from protein, which means about 52 grams per day for an average male and about 44 grams per day for an average female. But if you look at international standards, they are closer to 37 grams a day for an average male and 29 grams a day for an average female. The other point that is still being debated is how much complete protein and how much incomplete protein we need.

Many people believe they can only get protein from meat since it is a complete protein that has all the amino acids at high levels. Plant protein is called incomplete because although a single plant may have all the essential amino acids, it can be low in one or two of them when compared with a protein from most animal sources. However, this doesn't take the whole picture into account. Although a single vegetable protein does not contain all the amino acids you need, if you eat a combination of foods like nuts, seeds, cereals, lentils, and beans, you will get all the amino acids you need from the combination.

Also keep in mind that while lean and low-fat meat and poultry contain lots of protein, some meat and poultry also contain substances like growth hormones, antibiotics, and other things that might be harmful. Some nutritionists suggest that people should buy organic meats and poultry whenever possible, but these choices are often expensive. This is another area of nutrition where you will want to become more educated so you can make the best choices for yourself.

Fats

Believe it or not, your body needs a little bit of fat! There are three types of fatty acids, which together make up fat: saturated, polyunsaturated, and monounsaturated. Notice that I said "a little bit" of fat. Your total calories from fat for one day shouldn't be more than 20 percent of your daily calories and you have to make sure those calories are from the right combination of fats.

Saturated fatty acids are found mostly in meat (beef, veal, lamb, pork, and ham), dairy products (whole milk, cream, and cheese) some vegetable oils (coconut, palm kernel, shortening) and nuts and seeds such as walnuts and flax seeds. Saturated fats shouldn't make up more than 10 percent of your daily calories.

Polyunsaturated fatty acids are most plentiful in oils made from soybeans, safflowers, sunflowers, and corn. Polyunsaturated fats shouldn't make up more than 10 percent of your daily calories.

Monounsaturated fatty acids are found primarily in nuts and nut oils and butters and vegetable oils like olive, canola, and peanut. These fats shouldn't make up more than 10 to 15 percent of your daily calories.

Fish, nuts, and seeds have both monounsaturated and polyunsaturated fatty acids. Fish such as salmon, trout, and herring also contain a lot of omega-3 fatty acids, which many doctors and nutritionists say is very healthy for your cardiovascular system. (Some fish, however, such as tuna and swordfish, can contain high levels of mercury and should be eaten in moderation. If you are pregnant or nursing, you may want to avoid these.)

Your Nutrition Guidelines

There are a number of sources you can check out online that provide nutrition guidelines (see the resources section in the back of the book), but some people in the Winners' Circle swear by the individualized plan they got from the USDA mypyramid.gov Web site. (This site even has a special option for vegetarians.) Other members of the Winners' Circle say they worked with nutritionists to come up with a plan that's best for them, and a few say that eating a mostly raw food diet is the best change they've ever made. The idea of eating mostly raw food may not sound very appealing, but there are fantastic raw food restaurants popping up all over the place and the food is out of this world. You won't believe how gorgeous and delicious some of the choices on these menus are until you've seen them and tried them! When I first met Doug Caporrino, the nutritional expert and fitness guru for this book, he treated me to dinner at a raw food restaurant in Manhattan called Pure Food and Wine. I have to say I was blown away by how great everything was—including the no-fat, no-refined-sugar dessert that I had! (It did make me laugh, though, that food that was uncooked took so long to get to the table. I was wondering what the hell they were doing back there, but whatever it was it tasted delish!)

Doug says, "One of the most important things about nutrition is to stay as close to nature as possible. That means no artificial anything. As Jack La Lanne, first man of fitness and one of my greatest mentors, said, 'If man made it, I don't eat it.'" If you need to sweeten a food or drink, for example, use real cane sugar (not the white refined version of sugar), honey, or agave nectar.

Second, Doug says to try to eat organic food. It's often more expensive, but it's worth it. If you want to see the research, go to www.consumersunion.org. Doug says, "When you're buying fruits and vegetables look for the sticker with the SKU number on it. Any sticker beginning with the number 9 means it's organic. Any sticker beginning with the number 8 means it's genetically modified. Any other number means it is grown in the conventional manner with fertilizers and the possible use of chemicals."

Third, he suggests that you seriously consider reducing the amount of dairy that you eat. I've read pros and cons of eating and not eating dairy, so take the time to weigh the benefits and drawbacks and decide how much dairy you want or need.

Fourth, and possibly most important, drink more water! Doug says, "The daily rule of thumb is one quart for every fifty pounds of body weight, plus an additional ounce for every minute of cardio exercise that you do." He says when he tells people they probably need to drink more water, most of them tell him that they are already drinking a ton of it. But when they start keeping track, they find out that they're not even drinking half as much each day as they're supposed to. And have you ever noticed that the people with a bottle of water in their hand are often thin, but the people who are heavy are more likely to be drinking a diet soda? Makes you think!

DELIVER YOURSELF FROM TEMPTATION

How many loaves of raisin bread do you have to go through before you realize you can't buy raisin bread?

To stay in the maintenance game you must be as brutally honest as you can about the foods that you still have a very hard time eating in the proper portions. If you can come up with the top ten foods to keep out of your house, then boy do you have a real chance to keep the weight off! (If your mate or kids want these foods, tell them to eat them when they're not at home!) You can occasionally enjoy these foods as planned "treats" in single-size portions, but otherwise treat them like Superman treats kryptonite. Stay far away from them, because just being close to them is enough to make you weak! Willpower to me does not mean keeping foods around to prove you are strong enough to not eat them. To me, willpower means knowing yourself so well that you realize those foods should not be around and having the will to stand up for what you need and ask your family to live without your biggest temptations in the house or at least to live with less of them.

Okay, so here goes. I am going to be an example to you by showing you the bridges I have burned. After you read my list, take out your Winners' Circle Workbook and make your own list. You can probably easily come up with your top ten, but if there are a dozen or more, take the time to list them all.

Stacey's Top Ten Foods That Are Banned from the House!

1. Raisin bread or any other kind of bread.

2. Novelty ice creams—diet or regular—like ice cream sandwiches and bars. (They are too tempting and easy for me to go back for more.)
3. Candy of any kind.
4. Duck sauce in jars. (I must get it in the single packets that come with the takeout order.)
5. Cakes—diet or regular. (If I want to serve cake for company, I freeze one slice for myself for another time and send the rest of the cake home with my guests.)
6. Cookies—not even the diet ones, because my hand keeps going back for more. (If I have to have a cookie, I buy one low-fat cookie when I'm out.)
7. Frosting or cake mixes. (The one exception is No Pudge! brownies.)
8. Leftovers—except a single portion for the next day. (The rest are frozen in single-size portions for future meals.)
9. Soda! (I love diet soda, but if I bought it, I would drink a two-liter bottle in a day. If I want soda, I buy it in a single can when I'm out or I order it in a restaurant.)
10. Whipped cream—diet or regular. For some reason my mind tells me it's a "free" food!

Fun, Foolproof Fitness

Whether you have been exercising religiously, a few times a week, or sporadically, if you want to maintain your weight loss and get into (or stay in) shape, being consistent is critical to your success. Every single person who has been in the

Winners' Circle for more than five years makes exercise an important part of his or her life! If you haven't kept up a regular fitness routine in the past because it seemed like it would take too much time, energy, or both, you'll be happy to know that it doesn't have to be that time consuming or strenuous.

One way that people defeat themselves with exercise is they try to do too much too soon, decide that it's too difficult, and quit. If you've been exercising a few times a week, you can improve your fitness just by adding a few minutes onto your workout, or adding another day each week. If you're already working out every day, you can increase the intensity just a notch and get even more benefits, or you can add something simple like a twenty-minute walk with your dog or a friend a few times a week and enjoy getting into even better shape without much effort at all.

Your body functions best when you're doing exercises or playing sports that make your heart stronger (aerobic exercise), strengthen your bones and muscles (strength training), and stretch all of your muscles and your spine (flexibility training).

Finding exercises that you really enjoy and look forward to is a double victory! Make it part of your mission to keep trying different types of exercises and sports until you find two or three that you really like, because that will make it much easier to be consistent and keep it up. Recently a heavy friend of mine told me he decided to go back to ballet class—something he did in his teens that he loved. I was so impressed that he didn't let his size or age stop him. It's amazing how much more joy he gets from ballet class than from his gym. (Sometimes I put on my favorite music in my apartment and just dance. The more fun you can make it, the more you will do it.)

Some people despise exercise because they've heard the expression "no pain, no gain" and think it's true. It's not. Exercise should be physically engaging and demanding, and is often a little uncomfortable until you're in shape, but it should not be painful—at least not while you're doing it. The reason people sometimes feel sore after a workout is that lactic acid builds up in the muscles during exercise. Doug says, "That means your body is in an acidic state and the quicker you can get it back into an alkaline state, the better. The easiest way to do this is with fresh vegetable juice, made with carrots or some other vegetable that you like." If you begin gradually, though, and slowly build up your strength and endurance, the amount of soreness after you exercise should be minimal. Practicing flexibility exercises before and after you do a cardio or strength training session also helps to reduce muscle soreness. Taking a warm bath with Epsom salts or soaking in a hot tub for about ten minutes right after you exercise will help your body to deal with the excess lactic acid too. And it will feel damn great to boot! If exercise causes you to have muscle cramps, you may not be getting enough potassium or magnesium.

After you finish a workout session, you should feel a little physically tired, but also energized. You shouldn't be working out so intensely that you can barely make it up a flight of stairs after you've finished, or feel so wiped out that all you can do is lie on the couch the rest of the day. Athletes sometimes refer to the feeling after a good workout as "good tired." You can feel that you've put forth some effort and worked your muscles, but you also feel like you still have energy left over. People who are just beginning to get into a regular exercise routine are often amazed that they feel more energetic after they exercise than they felt beforehand. That's a great perk and one way you'll know if your workout is the right length and level of intensity for you.

How Much Exercise Do You Need to Maintain Your Weight?

To maintain your current weight, you need to "use up" as many calories during exercise as you eat each day. You burn some calories in the course of your normal day just by moving, but you probably don't work off nearly as many as you need to, unless you have a physically active job.

Figure out how much exercise you need to plan into your day:

1. Calculate your daily caloric intake by keeping track of what you eat each day, consulting a calorie counter, and adding up all your calories. The Web site www.caloriesperhour.com has a calculator that figures calories, protein, fat, carbohydrates, fiber, and sodium for over 23,200 foods from grocery stores, fast-food chains, and restaurants. (There are also reference books with many of these lists.)

2. Estimate how many calories you burn in a day without working out. Determine the calories burned during your daily activities and add them up to get your total. For instance, in a day you might walk a few blocks to work, run the vacuum, do the dishes, wash your car, or sweep the porch. (You use calories doing sedentary things like typing and reading too, but not very many!) To find out how many calories are burned in typical daily activities, look in a book that lists calorie counts for daily activities or use an online calculator such as www.primusweb.com/fitnesspartner/index.html.

3. Subtract the number of calories you naturally burn in a day from the number of calories you eat. The difference is the number of calories you need to burn each day with additional exercise to maintain your current weight. To do this very simply, take your current weight and add a zero to the end of it. If you weigh 140 pounds, your daily calorie intake should be around 1,400 to maintain your weight without exercise. Now, when you factor in exercise, you can go up some in calories or subtract some if you want to lose. (It's not an exact science but it's good enough for those of us who hate math!)

Add to Your Exercise Options

The exercise options listed below are from the Fitness Challenge game, which was one of *Health* magazine's Editor's Picks in 2005. Vicki Sorensen created the game to motivate herself and other "wannabe exercisers." A member of the Winners' Circle for going on five years, Vicki says, "I still don't love to exercise so I always have to coerce myself to do it. I find it difficult sometimes to prioritize exercise into my schedule. To this day, I really only exercise consistently when I have a partner playing the Fitness Challenge with me. I doubt that I'll ever be one of those people who jumps up in the morning and says, 'I can't wait to go exercise,' so finding a way to keep doing it consistently is very important for me and a battle that I'm determined to keep winning!"

Vicki's mother, Stephanie (Vicki's Fitness Challenge business partner), has maintained her weight loss for almost five years, mainly by consistently exercising. She says, "I was never the kind of person who automatically reaches for the fruit instead of the M&M's or the kind of person who jumps out of bed in the morning to run ten miles. So I used to rely on diets (I've tried them all!) to keep my weight down and probably lost at least 200 to 300 pounds over my adult life by crash dieting. I thought that unless you exercised until you couldn't breathe, you weren't doing yourself any good. I now know that moving as little as thirty to forty-five minutes at least three days a week can be very helpful. I walk three to four miles most mornings and take small walks during the day. Moving helps me eat better food and the right portions."

To calculate exactly how many calories you will burn doing each exercise, consult one of the online sites such as www.caloriesperhour.com. (If you type in "calorie burning calculator" in one of the search engines like Google, a list of free calculators will come up.)

To give you a ballpark estimate, though, Vicki says that the exercises on the Star-Studded list below burn an average of 300 calories per hour for someone who weighs about 130 pounds, and the options on the Star-Lite list burn less than 300 calories per hour for someone who weighs 130 pounds. These lists should help get you moving, or inspire you to try something new if you want to vary your workout.

Star-Studded
Aerobics (high impact)
Aerobics (step)
Basketball
Bicycling (outdoor and
   stationary)
Boxing
Calisthenics (push-ups,
   sit-ups)
Circuit training
Cross-country snow skiing
Dancing (ballet or modern)
Elliptical/cross-trainer
Football
Handball
Hiking
Jazzercise
Jogging/running

Judo, karate, kickboxing,
   tae kwon do
Kayaking
Lacrosse
Power walking
Racquetball
Rock climbing
Rollerblading/rollerskating
Rowing
Rugby
Snowshoeing
Soccer
Skipping rope
Squash
Stairmaster
Swimming
Tae bo
Tennis (singles)

Volleyball
Waterskiing
Weight lifting
Whitewater rafting

Star-Lite
Aerobics (low impact)
Badminton
Bowling
Canoeing
Frisbee
Golfing
Motocross
Paddleboat

Pilates
Skateboarding
Snowmobiling
Softball
Surfing
Tai chi
Tennis (doubles)
Unicycling
Volleyball
Walking
Water aerobics
Water volleyball
Yoga

Doug designed the following fitness plan so everyone can use it, including people who have knee or other joint challenges. The exercises are categorized under: cardiovascular, strength training, and flexibility training. This was very helpful to me because I need total knee replacement. It has been very hard to exercise as the knee gets worse. That puts me into panic mode, because if you don't move you cannot maintain unless you starve, and boy I know a lot better than to try that!

If you are just starting to exercise on a regular basis, follow the instructions for Beginners (and if you have physical issues, consult with your doctor before you get started). The Beginners' exercises can also be helpful if you've gotten off track of your regular routine. If you're already in shape, follow the instructions for Athletes. You may already have your own fitness regimen that's working well for you. If so, great! You might still want to add some of these exercises to your repertoire, though particularly if you want to beef up your efforts in one of the three categories.

Cardiovascular Training

The key to cardio training is monitoring your heart rate. A heart rate monitor and a pedometer that counts steps are the best pieces of equipment you can own. Until you can get a heart rate monitor, there is a basic formula you can use to determine what your heart rate should be for a healthy cardiovascular workout.

Basic Formula to Determine Maximum Heart Rate for Exercising

Subtract your age from the number 220. Then take 70 percent of that number and the total will give you an idea of what your maximum heart rate should be while doing cardiovascular exercise.

How to Determine Your Heart Rate While Exercising
1. Stop and take your pulse by gently pressing on the side of your neck (the carotid pulse).
2. Beginning with zero, count the number of beats for six seconds. (Count the first beat as zero.)
3. Multiply the number you get by 10 to find out the average number of times your heart is beating per minute.

Basically, when you're doing aerobic exercises, you should feel a little out of breath, but not be so winded that you can't talk. When you're getting a good workout, you will probably break a sweat, but you can't go by that alone because the amount each person perspires is different and the weather obviously has an effect too. If you're swimming, you can be sweating and not even know it.

Do the following exercises (or your own choice of cardio exercise) at least three times a week. If you choose an exercise not listed in the examples below, you can still follow the guidelines for Beginners or Athletes to give you an idea of how much you should start with and what you should be working up to.

Walking, Jogging, or Cycling

Walking, jogging, and riding a bike are all excellent cardio exercises.

Beginners

Start by walking or cycling just 10 minutes a day. At the end of one week, increase your time to 15 minutes. After two weeks, increase the time to 20 minutes. At the beginning of week four, increase your time to 30 minutes. Continue doing 30 minutes each time until it starts to feel easy. Then consider increasing that time by 10 minutes or so each week until you reach the duration that allows you to burn as many calories as you want to burn.

Athletes

Start by walking or cycling 30 minutes a day. At the end of one week, increase your time to 35 minutes. At the beginning of the third week, increase your time to 40 minutes. Continue doing 40 minutes each time until it starts to feel easy. Then increase that time by 10 minutes each week until you reach the duration that allows you to burn as many calories as you want to burn.

Swimming

If walking, running, or cycling puts too much stress on your joints, or you just love the feeling of being in water, try swimming. Working out in the water protects your joints from pressure so you can get your heart rate up and burn calories without pain. Many health clubs and fitness centers also have kickboards, so you can float your upper body while letting your hips and legs do most of the work. Some pools also have floats to put between your calves or ankles, for when you want to give your upper body a better workout. If the pool where you swim offers swimming classes, consider taking a class or two to learn more strokes or improve the form and efficiency of the strokes you already know.

Beginners and Athletes

Weeks one and two: Swim the number of laps that it takes you to feel out of breath. (If you are winded after one lap, that's okay. It's a good starting point.)

March or jog in place at the shallow end of the pool until you catch your breath. Then swim the same number of laps you began with.

Alternate swimming laps with marching or jogging in place for a total of 10 to 15 minutes if you are a Beginner and for 20 to 30 minutes if you are an Athlete.

Week three: Follow the instructions for weeks one and two, but increase your total time by 5 minutes if you are a Beginner and by 10 minutes if you are an Athlete.

Week four: Continue the same routine, but increase your time by another 5 minutes, so Beginners are working out for a total of 20 to 25 minutes and Athletes are working out for a total of 35 to 45 minutes.

Week five: Increase the number of consecutive laps you are swimming by one lap if you're a Beginner and by two laps if you're an Athlete.

Week six: Increase the number of laps you swim in between marching or jogging in place until you are able to swim continuously for 20 to 30 minutes if you are a Beginner and for 35 to 45 minutes if you are an Athlete. When you reach that level of ability, begin and end your workouts by jogging or marching in place for 3 to 5 minutes for a good warm-up and cooldown. This will give you an excellent cardio workout!

Strength Training

In strength training exercise, a form of resistance, like free weights, weight machines, or exercise resistance bands, is used to strengthen your muscles. You should do 2 to 3 non-consecutive strength training sessions each week. The duration of each session will depend on the number of sets and repetitions you are doing.

Warm-up: Before doing any of the strength training exercises below, warm up your muscles for 5 to 7 minutes by jumping rope, walking, jogging in place, or doing jumping jacks.

Cooldown: After these exercises, cool down your muscles for 5 to 7 minutes by doing slow static stretching (hold a stretch for 20 to 30 seconds, no bouncing) and practicing deep breathing (inhale for 6 seconds, hold for 6 seconds, and exhale for 6 seconds).

Arm Curls

Beginners

1. Stand with your feet shoulder width apart, your legs straight without locking your knees, and your back straight.
2. Holding hand weights that are 2 to 5 pounds each, extend your arms straight out in front of you, with your palms facing the ceiling. (If you don't have hand weights, look in your pantry for soup cans or plastic

bottles of sauces or salad dressing. Keep in mind that 16 oz. of contents equals about one pound.

3. Keeping your upper arms parallel with the floor and bending at the elbow, bring the weights toward you until they almost touch your shoulders, then bring them back to the original position.

4. For the first two weeks, do one set of 10 repetitions. During the third and fourth weeks, do two sets of 10 repetitions. Beginning the fifth week, do three sets of 10 to 15 repetitions. Once three sets of 10 to 15 repetitions feels comfortable, start over from the beginning but follow the instructions for Athletes.

Athletes

Follow the same instructions for Beginners, except:

Use hand weights that are 5 or 10 pounds.
Do two sets of 10 repetitions for the first two weeks.
During the third and fourth weeks, do two sets of 15 repetitions.
Beginning the fifth week, do three sets of 15 repetitions.

Leg Extensions

Beginners

1. Sit in a straight-back chair with your feet flat on the floor and shoulder width apart.

2. Extend your right leg so it is straight (but the knee is not locked).

3. Bend your right knee so your foot returns to the floor.

4. Repeat this movement 12 to 15 times to make one set.

5. Switch to the left leg and follow the same instructions.

During weeks one and two, do one set on each leg. During weeks three and four, do two sets. Beginning on week five, follow the instructions for Athletes.

Athletes

Begin with three sets of 15 repetitions. After two weeks, wear a pair of 5-pound or 10-pound ankle weights to increase the level of difficulty or do the leg extensions on a weight machine with 5 or 10 pounds. You can continue adding more weight over time, until you can lift 20 pounds per leg for three sets of 15 to 20 repetitions. (Do not add more weight unless you want to build muscle bulk.)

Limb Stretch and Lift

This exercise strengthens your back muscles. You should not do it if you have skeletal-related back problems.

Beginners

1. Lie flat on the floor on your stomach, with your arms out in front of you and your palms touching the floor.

2. Lift your arms and legs an inch or so off the floor.

3. Hold for 3 to 5 seconds and then slowly lower your arms and legs back to the floor.

4. Let your entire body relax for a count of 5 seconds and then repeat.

(Begin by doing this exercise 3 to 5 times in a row and work up to doing it 10 to 12 times. Once you are comfortably able to do this exercise 12 times in a row, follow the instructions for Athletes.)

Athletes

Follow the same instructions for Beginners, but hold the position for 10 to 20 seconds before lowering your arms and legs back to the floor.

Backward Leg Lifts

Beginners

1. Lie on the floor on your stomach with your arms and hands down at your side.

2. While keeping your legs straight, lift them off of the floor as high as you comfortably can and hold for 5 to 10 seconds. (If lifting or holding up both legs at once is too difficult, lift only one leg at a time until you are strong enough to lift them together.)

3. Slowly lower your legs (or leg) back to the floor.

4. Repeat this motion 10 times to complete one set.

5. Work up to three sets of 10 repetitions. (After you have done three sets of 10 repetitions for three weeks, follow the instructions for Athletes.)

Athletes

Follow the same instructions for Beginners, but hold your legs up for 20 to 30 seconds.

Once you have established a basic strength training routine, consider varying or increasing your routine by mixing in other exercises, such as sit-ups, push-ups, pull-ups, leg presses, and bench presses.

Flexibility Training

You will get the most benefit from flexibility training by stretching your muscles for at least 10 to 15 minutes four or five days a week, whether or not your exercise for the day includes a cardio workout or strength training. The best-case scenario is to make flexibility training part of your day *every* day.

Flexibility is very important for keeping your muscles and joints healthy and maintaining your mobility. Not only that, but once stretching becomes a part of your daily routine, you'll discover how great it feels. We all hold tension in our muscles and sometimes we don't even realize how tight we are until we start to stretch.

Doug Caporrino says, "Your stretching will have the greatest benefits if it is slow and steady. You should never bounce to extend your stretching. This ultimately makes your muscles tighter and does more harm than good. Your objective is to stretch as far as your body will allow (without causing pain) and hold the stretch for 20 to 30 seconds while deeply and slowly inhaling through your nose and exhaling through your mouth (this is called *static* stretching). Try to balance the length of your inhalations and exhalations by making each one last for 6 to 8 seconds. Each time you exhale your body will become more relaxed and eventually take you further and further in the stretch."

The following stretches are for both Beginners and Athletes.

Full Leg Stretch

1. Sit on the floor as if you are sitting in a straight-backed chair.
2. Gently lean forward, keeping your back straight, and attempt to touch your ankles. (Only go as far as you can without curving your back.)
3. Hold the stretch for 20 to 30 seconds (and remember to breathe).
4. Repeat this stretch three times.

Hamstring Stretch

1. Lie flat on the floor on your back.
2. Keeping your right leg straight, lift it into the air as far as you can without bending your knee.

3. Grasp the back of your thigh with both hands and gently pull your leg toward your chest. Hold for 20 seconds.
4. Repeat this three times.
5. Repeat steps 1–4 with your left leg.

Arm Stretch

1. Stand straight with your feet shoulder width apart.
2. Put both hands behind you with your palms touching.
3. Clasp your hands together, intertwining your fingers.
4. Lift your clasped hands up and away from your back, while keeping your back straight.
5. Hold for 20 to 30 seconds (and remember to breathe).
6. Relax your arms back down to your sides and gently shake them out.
7. Repeat steps 1–6 three times.

Incorporate Exercise into Your Daily Life

People often think of exercise as a solo activity, but there are a lot of ways to do it with others and make moving part of your daily life, so you're not relying totally on your regular exercise routine or visits to the gym. Look into community sports teams and recreational facilities that offer opportunities to play softball, volleyball, basketball, tennis, badminton, soccer, flag football, or water polo. You can also join forces with one or more people to play sports together or to exercise together. One way to do that is by playing the Fitness Challenge game (see the resources section for more details). Walk with a friend in the mall on rainy days, and most important, stop looking for the closest spots when you park your car to go shopping. Park in the last space—I guarantee if you do this all the time you will see a big difference in yourself.

You can also re-create your social outings to be more active. Instead of meeting friends for dinner or a drink, meet them for a walk through the park or a game of tennis, golf, or another sport you all enjoy. The next time you plan a party, think fun and action instead of food and drinks! Do something original like inviting your friends to go bowling or on a bike ride. Don't make food the center of the event; make it secondary. There are lots of great options if you use your creativity and keep an open mind!

Balancing Improvement with Acceptance

Amy Ojerholm explains that to make a winning maintenance plan, you need to strike a balance between making changes and accepting the reality of things that can't be changed. She says, "Everyone is struggling to live as well as they can and because we're all dealt cards that we can't control, it's unrealistic to expect anything in our lives to be perfect all the time." (I personally have made up my mind that I am no longer going to feel sorry for myself about the cards I've been dealt.

Instead, I'm gonna make the best card game you ever laid eyes on!)

The first step toward finding a balance between change and acceptance is knowing you have limitations and acknowledging that you've done the best you could in the past. Amy says, "If the only message you ever give yourself is 'change, change, change,' you're going to have a hard time doing that because you're not going to feel like anything you've done thus far deserves any credit. And then you're going to get burned out and depleted and feel terrible about yourself. That's why it's so important to recognize that you've done the best you could so far and that whatever you've accomplished, no matter how small you may think it is, has value. You have to accept that even the things that you've done wrong in the past have merit because they were the methods you adopted in order to cope with stress and survive." It was the best thing you could do with the information you had at the time.

The second step to achieving a sense of balance between improvement and acceptance is being honest about the areas of your life in which you most want to grow. Amy says, "Being aware of the behaviors and situations that you want to improve is important because if all you do is accept that you've done the best you could and settle for that, you won't make any forward progress in your life and that will eventually make you feel bad about yourself too." It might help if you think of this back-and-forth between change and acceptance like a seesaw or teeter-totter. Some days you're in acceptance mode and some days you're in change mode and ideally the seesaw will be somewhat balanced.

The way to experience the most success in your growth is to do it in small steps instead of trying to do it all at once. It's important to do what you can instead of getting upset about what you can't do. For example, if you're not physically fit enough to run, commit to walking and remind yourself that improvement in this area doesn't have to be running. You can continue to improve by walking longer or walking faster or walking more often. When I first started exercising I bought a pedometer that counted steps so I could see my progress. The first day I could hardly walk ten steps. But within a week, I could walk from the front door of my building to the mailbox and back. Within a few weeks, I could walk a block. Every day my goal was just to walk a few more steps, and now I walk miles without even thinking about it. Just remember to step it up every day.

Write Your Own Script

To make a winning game plan and be able to stick with it, you have to be willing to take charge of your day in a way that you may not be used to doing. Dr. Greer says that writing your script puts you completely in charge of your day. She explains, "Instead of allowing other people and outside forces to shape your choices, take the proactive approach of making smart decisions for yourself ahead of time. This puts you in total control of your actions." The way to begin practicing this is to sit down and make a Do List for yourself. This list will include two or three things that you know are good for you, mentally and emotionally, that you will do each day.

She says, "Keep in mind that this *isn't* a to-do list. To-do lists tend to include items that you have to do or think you should do. While those things are often important to complete, they rarely give you the same sense or satisfaction that you get from planning and doing the things you most enjoy. Your Do List is exclusively for activities that you want to do and love to do!"

Dr. Greer explains that you can make a Do List that's different for each day, or you can make one that you'll use for several days, a week, or more. That's entirely up to you. The idea is to teach yourself how to make fulfilling choices and follow through with them. For example, your Do List might say: (1) Start the day with affirmations, (2) Dance to three songs, (3) Read five pages of an inspiring or funny book. Next to each item on your list, write down why that choice is important to you and how following through with the choice will benefit you.

"Your objective," says Dr. Greer, "is to develop the internal control to formulate and implement the choices that are in your best interest. In order to do that you really need to invest the mental energy and time in yourself to think about what's most important to you, what your highest priorities are, and what you plan to achieve and actualize each day. This will increase your self-awareness a thousandfold. People who have struggled with overeating often overload their schedules in the same way that they used to overload themselves with food. The key to successfully writing your own script is to keep it manageable by only putting a few items on your Do List for each day. Just as you're learning to enjoy a taste or a few bites of sweets or high-calorie foods instead of eating the whole cake, you're learning how to indulge in bite-size portions of rewarding activities that make you feel good."

She stresses that it's also important to remember that this is *not* a "Don't List"! She says, "When you're making your Do List, always focus on what you want to experience or accomplish that is positive. That way, every item on your list becomes a building block to self-esteem and success. By giving time and attention to your Dos, the Don'ts will take care of themselves. Essentially, the more energy you invest in making plans and choices that are good for you, the less time and energy you have for doing things that aren't. Writing your own script makes you aware of what you most want to say yes to in your life."

Take out your Winners' Circle Workbook and make your first Do List now. Use this list as your model for future lists. Also decide whether you want to make a different list each day, each week, or just when the spirit moves you! For ideas of what to include in your Do Lists, refer back to Dr. Nadler's advice earlier in the chapter under "Plan to Win." You might want to make a master list of possibilities so you always have a mental health menu to choose from. It will also be fun for you to keep adding to that list and watching it grow and seeing yourself cross off all your accomplishments.

Make Plans, Not Excuses

You may have heard the expressions you can't con a con artist or you can't kid a kidder. When it comes to excuses, I've heard them all and used most of them myself. I'm not a doctor or a psychologist, but I could have a PhD in excuses! So if it feels like I'm being hard on you in this book, it's just my way of trying to nudge you out of denial and into being real with yourself. Whether you will win at keeping the excess weight off comes down to one simple fact: either you want to maintain your current weight or you are looking for reasons to gain it back.

Every excuse you feed yourself will eventually lead to a pound and then two and then ten or more. If maintaining your weight is truly as important as you say it is, you need to come up with at least two ways to deal with every excuse that you hear yourself say.

Sit down right now, open your Winners' Circle Workbook, and make a list of the excuses you use over and over again. (And don't use the excuse that you're too busy to make the list!) Beneath each excuse, write down two or more ways to outsmart the excuse. Here are some examples:

I have to keep cookies and candy in the house for my kids
1. Your children will be much healthier without the fat and sugar. If you want to give them the best you can offer, give them fruit snacks and low-fat and low-sugar choices that you can also eat.

2. If you really believe your kids will be worse off without the sugar rush and the fatty snacks, buy them one cookie or piece of candy at a time while you're out with them. This approach will teach them to savor the treat and help them to learn moderation. Or you can give them money for the ice cream man. Help them to learn the truth about a single-size portion.

I can't afford a gym right now

1. You were always able to come up with the money to buy the food you used to overindulge in, so if you really want to join a gym you can find a way to arrange your budget to support that choice. There are many gyms and Ys that offer scholarships or will let you pay according to your income. Check it out.

2. You don't have to belong to a gym to get a good workout. You can walk around your neighborhood, inside a shopping mall, or if you live in an apartment building, you might even be able to walk back and forth on your roof. (Some days I take the elevator in my building down to the lobby and walk back up to my apartment on the twelfth floor. That is a free and fast way to get your heart rate up.) You can check out exercise books, videos, and DVDs at your local library for free.

Because of my job or schedule I have to eat out a lot

You can order something low-fat and at least relatively healthy in just about any restaurant in the country. If you find yourself at a hot-dog or hamburger joint, that doesn't mean you have a reason to go hog wild! Opt for a salad and get your meat without the bun. Use mustard or ketchup and relish instead of mayo or high-fat condiments or dressings. Many of the people in the Winners' Circle have jobs that involve traveling and spend many evenings in restaurants with clients or in hotel dining rooms by themselves. They all agree that dining out doesn't equal weight gain unless you ignore your game plan.

Winners' Wisdom to Beat the Odds

Use the Method of Measurement That Works Best for You

To weigh every day or not to weigh every day, that is the question. The Winners' Circle is split down the middle on this question. About half of them weigh themselves every morning, while the other half use other measurements, like how their clothes fit, or having their body fat tested once a month. They all agree, though, that you need to pick a way to stay totally in touch with your size and weight and stick with the method you choose. There's some pretty compelling research that shows that once people who have lost weight gain some of it back—even as few as seven to ten pounds—it can be very difficult to lose it again. Some of the latest studies show that people who weigh themselves daily have a better chance of maintaining their goal weight.

For example, Margaret—one of the daily-weighing advocates—said, "I'm only four feet nine inches, so even a few pounds makes a big difference in how I feel and how I look. I don't want the extra weight to sneak up on me, so I weigh myself every day. If I notice that I've put on more than a pound or two and I know it's not water weight, that tells me I have to be more careful about what I'm eating for a couple weeks and increase my exercise a little. Losing a couple pounds every once in a while is easy. I just don't want to be surprised by getting on the scale and seeing that I've gained five or more pounds, because that would mean being really careful for more than a month to take it back off and I don't want to go through that."

People like Margaret know that the scale can go up or down a couple pounds and they don't get elated or depressed by those varying numbers. But if they see that the scale has gone up more than a few pounds, they know they need to exercise a little more and make better food choices.

Patrick, on the other hand, who has been in the Winners' Circle for more than ten years, says he only weighs himself if his clothes feel a little tight. When he gets on the scale, if he's gained a few pounds, he immediately does what it takes to lose them again.

A big part of maintenance is being honest and being willing to face the truth, whatever it is. So be honest with yourself about how you should monitor your weight and size and be faithful about keeping up your chosen method. If you find yourself obsessively weighing (more than once a day), it is a clear sign of danger ahead.

Tips of Wisdom from the Winners' Circle

Joanne—Practice portion control. Learn the size or weight of a single serving of all the foods you typically eat.

Helen—Prepare food when you're not hungry.

Nick—Remember that it takes twenty minutes for your brain to know you're full. Before you let yourself have a second helping, wait at least twenty minutes.

Yvonne—Once a month, let yourself splurge on a food you don't usually allow yourself to eat.

Vicki—Snack throughout the day to keep your energy level consistent so you never get too hungry. Keep quick, healthy snack staples at the ready. For treats, label them as "calorie-worthy" or not, to help you decide whether you really want to eat them.

Stephanie—Avoid elastic waistbands so you know exactly when you put on a few pounds.

Emily—If you have a dog, walk it! Not only is it good exercise for you and the canine you love, it is a good motivator to do something the dog will appreciate.

Sherry—Don't say, or even think, the words "I can't."

Stacey—Remove the words "I blew it" from your vocabulary and replace them with the words "I'm done." Do not bring piles of Tupperware to your friends' dinner parties so you can take home leftovers. (I swear I did that all the time and I wasn't even embarrassed!)

Plan Your Success!

Now that you've read what the experts say and gotten some great advice from the Winners' Circle, it's time to take out your Winners' Circle Workbook and write your plan.

Make Your Food Plan

For your food plan, make an Optimum Nutrition List. Using the categories of carbohydrates, protein, and fats covered earlier in the chapter, list the choices for each that you know are best for you. Under each category, also include foods that you're curious about but haven't tried yet, like exotic fruits or vegetables, different types of whole grains like millet, amaranth, or teff, and maybe some soy products like tofu. (Check out some of the cookbooks listed in the resources section to help you expand your horizons!)

Manage and Monitor Your Nutrition

Decide how you are going to manage and monitor your food each day. Write down what method you will be using. (Some of the possibilities include keeping a food journal, counting calories and/or fat grams, and measuring portions.) When you have been successfully maintaining for a year or so (for some people it's less time, for others much longer), you will be able to eyeball the right portions, but wait until you are clearly ready. When you find yourself overeating, go back to a more rigid monitoring system for a while.

Meal Planning

Write down how many meals you will eat each day and how you will ensure that the meals are healthy and made up of items from your Optimum Nutrition List.

Snacks

Decide whether or not you are going to include snacks in your game plan. If so, decide and write down how many snacks you will have each day and make a list of snacks (including portion size or total calories) that you can choose from.

Make Your Fitness Plan

Make your Optimum Fitness List. Under the primary fitness categories, list all of your top choices. Decide and write down how much exercise you are going to do each day. Be sure that your exercise plan includes aerobic exercise, strength training, and flexibility training. And if you are physically challenged, do all you are capable of doing. Even people in wheelchairs can get their heart rates up. If you don't move it you might lose it. I not only believe that, but have seen it with my own eyes.

Manage and Monitor Your Fitness

Decide and describe how you are going to manage and monitor your fitness. Will you be keeping track of the calories you burn, keeping track of the amount of minutes you exercise, noting the mileage, laps, or number of repetitions you do? (I look at the lengths of the songs on my favorite music CDs and add up the minutes of all the songs. That way, if I walk for five songs I know exactly how long I was walking. I started with two songs and then three, and now I walk to the whole CD.) Whatever method or methods you use to keep track, it's a good idea to make a section in your Winner's Circle Workbook to record your progress or possibly keep a separate exercise log. It's very rewarding to look back and see how much you've done and how much you've improved!

Decide and write down when you will exercise each day. Some members of the Winners' Circle swear by starting each day with some form of exercise, while others prefer to take a fitness break in the middle of the day or right after work. If you don't already know the time of day that's best for you, try each of the suggestions for one week, and see which one feels best.

THE IMPERFECT TEN

The Top Ten *Worst* Reasons for Not Making a Winning Game Plan

1. I don't have time. (Get real!)
2. I think it's better to be spontaneous. (I spontaneously got to 550 pounds.)
3. I can't decide what to do. (Did you decide to be fat?)

4. I'm waiting until I feel inspired to do it. (Keep waiting.)

5. I'll be able to make a plan after I move. (There is no such thing as a geographical location cure. You take your challenges with you wherever you go!)

6. It's too expensive. (Hospitals and funerals are far more expensive.)

7. I'll make a plan when the weather gets better. (Your game plan isn't seasonal! You have to be able to win in all weather.)

8. I don't have anyone to support me in this venture. I can't go it alone. (No, you can't. But a support team isn't going to show up at your door. Seeking them out is when your recovery officially begins. Trust me on this one.)

9. I can't give up my favorite food forever! (You don't have to. Remember, nobody got obese eating an occasional doughnut or two. It was the "dozens" that did us in.)

10. I can't do it until after the holidays.

Sounds like you haven't looked at a calendar lately . . .
    September—Labor Day and Jewish holidays
    October—Halloween
    November—Thanksgiving
    December—Christmas and Chanukah
    January—New Year's

February—Valentine's Day
March—St. Patrick's Day
April—Passover and Easter
May—Mother's Day, Memorial Day
June—Father's Day
July—Independence Day

That leaves August for getting your winning plan in order, and remember that shrinks go on vacation in August, so good luck!

STEP 3

·········

Turn Pain into Power
Use It to Lose It

*Except for our own thoughts, there is nothing absolutely
in our power.*

—René Descartes, *A Discourse on Method*

Most people swear they would do anything to get rid of their emotional pain. Whether your pain is from heartache, unresolved issues or events from your past, the new challenges and problems that you're facing now, or all of these, you probably wish you could avoid it or get over it. But emotional pain is as much a part of life as pleasure and happiness. As long as you're alive, you're going to have to deal with it. The questions are, how much and how long are you going to let it make you suffer?

The truth, strange as it sounds, is that the more pain you have, the more power you can have if you're willing to turn the pain into the fuel you need to do the things you care about. Try thinking of the sadness, fear, guilt, regret, and other negative emotions that you have as "growing pains." Each new hurdle that you jump earns you another notch on your bedpost of life! There is an amazing amount of freedom and power that comes from knowing you can work through and overcome pain instead of running away from it or numbing yourself with food.

Step 3 teaches you how to turn your pain into power by healing the heartache and resolving the issues that are stopping you from living your life to its fullest. You will find out why the pain doesn't disappear with the pounds, how to get comfortable with your new size, how to introduce the people you care about to the new you, and how making new friends can add freedom to your life. You will learn what you can do to cope with your regrets, begin accepting the things you can't change, and learn a dozen different ways to empower yourself. For those of you who are struggling with body image issues (who isn't?) this chapter includes a special section on getting more comfortable in your own skin— literally. So you can put that new comfort level to good use, you'll find out how to crank up your sexual joy meter and create the connection you crave. (Yee-ha!)

The Pain Doesn't Disappear with the Pounds

You probably already know that losing weight isn't a magical solution for all of your problems and doesn't eliminate the reasons that led to your being overweight in the first place. Whatever made you want to overeat will affect you until you face it and resolve it, or at least learn how to manage it. You can't maintain if you can't face the pain. For most people, becoming thinner creates some new challenges. Now that you've lost weight, you probably don't have friends and family cheering you on to keep it off, like they were when you were initially losing it. When you were heavier, you may have thought that if only you could be thin, life would be fabulous and you would be ecstatically happy. But the reality—after you take off the rose-colored glasses—is that the emotional pain comes up when you put the food down.

You have to feel the emotional pain now, and if you want to maintain your weight, you have to work through these things or they will never really go away and your pounds will not stay away. They'll always be there haunting you. The upside is that every time you face something big, it's a little easier than the time before because you know the pain's not going to last forever. You can also learn new ways to deal with the pain that are healthy instead of self-destructive. The key is to figure out what you need to do and what works for you.

There's no doubt that losing weight and the changes that go with keeping it off have an effect on your relationships. Some of them get better, others get worse, and some end altogether. What makes this even trickier is that what you expect to happen and what really happens are usually different. Sometimes very different!

For example, some people in the Winners' Circle said they thought losing weight would improve the relationships they had with their parents. Most of these people said their parents gave them a hard time about their weight and criticized them for not having more self-discipline or not taking better care of themselves, so they thought losing weight would win their parents' approval and maybe even praise. But in most of these situations, either their parents downplayed their accomplishments or found other things to criticize. For the most part, whatever type of relationship they had with their parents when they were heavy continued to be the kind of relationship they had after they lost weight.

Many people in the Winners' Circle said they thought their spouses or significant others would find them more attractive and desirable after they lost weight. Some of their partners *did* increase their attention and affection and want sex more often, but a lot of them said, "I love you the same now as I did before."

A lot of the single people said they thought they'd have an easier time meeting new people and would be going out on more dates. Other singles thought that being thinner would lead to a meaningful relationship or help them to find and attract their soul mate. Some of the single women and men are dating more and some of them are in meaningful relationships, but they don't think being a smaller size in itself is what made the difference. Several of them said that having more self-respect, self-esteem, and confidence made it easier for them to meet new people and that the lessons they learned as they were losing weight helped them to be more open and accepting with other people.

One woman said, "When I lost weight, I had seventeen first dates in a row. Men were attracted to me, but they never called back for a second date. When I was fat I always said the men who didn't ask me out or didn't call back were shallow and not mature enough to see beyond my weight. But after seventeen guys in a row didn't call me back when I was a size 8, I had to take another look at myself. On the inside, not the outside. I finally did what my best friends tried to get me to do for years. I found a therapist and started working on all the shit that I went through with my father. It sounds so Freudian it's embarrassing, but the year I've spent in therapy has been worth a million dollars. When I let myself see what I was doing and how I behaved, it was no wonder nobody asked me on a second date! I'm still not in a serious relationship. I'm not really ready for that, but I'm having fun dating and I'm not scaring men away anymore."

For people who rarely or never dated until after they lost weight, the feeling of being naked without the "invisibility cloak" of extra pounds along with feeling like a fish out of water can make for some pretty uncomfortable situations. After losing most of my weight I started dating for the first time in my life. Hey, it was a little late in the game, but at least I was in the game. When I went on my first few dates I sucked at it. I did not know how to act on a date so I thought back to high school and decided to go on my next few dates pretending to be Dawny Benson. Dawny was talented and beautiful and every girl wanted to be her, including me, so that was my great plan for when I went out on my first few dates. I would act how I thought Dawny would act on a date. And I had the nerve to wonder why the hell those dates went bad! Ha! I acted like a giddy seventeen-year-old moron, flipping my hair and giggling at bad jokes. I hid my best quality from each date, which has always been and still is my personality! Live and learn.

The bottom line is that losing weight doesn't solve the relationship problems that you had when you were heavier and it doesn't magically give you experience and abilities that you didn't already have. But it can give you a new lease on life so you can work through the old problems, learn how to handle the new ones, and keep improving yourself one step at a time.

Introduce Family and Old Friends to the New You!

Most of the people who successfully maintain their goal weight say that the changes that took place on the inside are at least as dramatic as the ones on the outside. They think differently, they feel differently, and in some cases their philosophy of life is different too. But since other people—even the ones you're close to—can't read your mind, it will be up to you to introduce them to the new person that you're becoming. Be warned, this will take patience and perseverance, because once people have an idea of who you are in their mind, it's hard to change that even if you live with them or see them every day. Sometimes that actually makes it harder. So the first thing you have to do is accept that very few people will notice the changes you're making on the inside until they have a chance to see over and over again the new choices you make and the new ways you behave. Don't try to prove anything to them; just be your new self and one day they will get it.

No matter how much you grow and change, some of your family members and old friends will probably still see you and treat you as the old you. It's been years since I've stayed in bed past 10 a.m., but I still get phone messages from people saying, "I know you're still in bed, but give me a call this afternoon when you're up." Meanwhile, by the time I get the message I have already walked my dog, gone swimming, and done some errands. Even after I've explained my new schedule to these people, their memory of how things used to be is their reality. Some of them will eventually catch up with the new you, and to help the others along, try to keep a sense of humor and make a game of it.

Instead of telling them new things about yourself or how your opinions or choices have changed, get them to play a version of the guessing game. You can say, "I had lunch at the diner today and guess what I ordered?" Or, "Guess what time I got up today?" Or tell them about something you saw on TV or witnessed in person that would have really upset you in the past, and then say, "Guess what I thought when I saw that?" Getting them engaged in learning about the changes you've made will help the new reality to sink in. Most people are much more likely to remember what they say than what you tell them. So if they're guessing what you ordered at the diner and eventually hit on "salad" and you say, "Yes! You win the prize!" that has a better chance of sinking in than if you say, "Hey, I went to the diner today and instead of having a cheeseburger I had a salad."

I'm grateful for my old friends because they help me remember where I came from, and I'm grateful to my new friends because they help me to forget where I came from. Your new friends give you a chance to practice being the new you because the new you is all they know. New friendships offer you the freedom to move forward and practice your new behaviors and choices without having to explain anything, defend yourself, or be reminded of what you used to do.

For the most part, people treat you the way you teach them and allow them to treat you. So one of the best ways to behave with old friends and new friends alike is to treat yourself the way you want them to treat you. If you want them to respect you, you have to respect yourself. If you want them to avoid criticizing you, don't criticize yourself. If you want them to see that you have self-worth, treat yourself in a way that shows you value yourself. For example, using and enjoying your material possessions is a clear sign that you value yourself. This life is too short not to use your good handbags or wear your best suits, even if you live a hundred years. I used to put my good things away for when my life was just the way I thought it should be, but not anymore. By using your good dishes, wearing your nice clothes and jewelry, and enjoying the finer things in life, you reinforce the idea that you deserve the best and you communicate that message to others.

Don't Let One Addiction Lead to Another

Dealing with the pain of your past means finding other ways to satisfy your needs without replacing overeating with other destructive behaviors. Some recovering alcoholics and drug addicts get hooked on food and get fat, some become sex addicts, and some sex addicts turn to alcohol and drugs. They should have all those recovery meetings in one big building so people could just move from one room to the next. Frankly, when I saw the coffee, doughnuts, and bowls of sugar cubes provided at AA, I sort of wished I could have been attending those meetings instead of Overeaters Anonymous! But in my case, stealing was the new behavior du jour (I still think in food terms). When I first lost weight, I hadn't found a healthy replacement for the food yet, so the need to act out in some way and keep my life filled with drama was very strong. That is, until the day I got more drama than I bargained for and a decade's worth of embarrassment to boot!

It was a cold winter day, but the sun was shining and I was feeling antsy. I dressed to the nines, did my makeup, and put on my baby blue suede coat. My matching gloves, sunglasses, and oversized leather handbag completed my Madison Avenue mystique. I grabbed my keys and left my apartment, needing and anticipating the thrill of adventure. I walked to a neighborhood grocery store, then strolled through the aisles putting a few food items that I needed into my shopping cart and nonchalantly slipping some shampoo, eye shadow, lipstick, and Aleve into my leather bag. My heart beat faster from the excitement.

As I was standing in line at the checkout counter, the store's security guard walked up to me and said, "I saw you take that shampoo. Please step over here with me and empty your bag. When he discovered the other items I had stolen he asked me for my ID and typed the information into a computer. I desperately tried to figure a way out of this mess but even I (a.k.a. Ms. Milton Bradley) had run out of games. When he confirmed that I wasn't on the most wanted list, he asked me to sign a form saying I would never again enter that store or any store in that chain. If I did, I would be arrested on the spot. Just as I was wondering how in the hell they would ever know it was me if I came in again, he took a Polaroid camera out of his desk and asked me to stand against the wall so he could take my picture. Half of the people in the store were already watching this drama play out, and when the flash went off it caught the attention of the other half. I vowed to get it together and never steal again, and I haven't. The thing is that if I had made a game plan for myself and found other forms of pleasure to fill the gap that food used to fill, that would never have happened. I wasn't stealing because I needed the stuff I put into my bag; I was doing it for the adrenaline rush. I still shop more than I need to, but now I pay for everything!

Turning pain into power is an ongoing process, and until the pain is gone you have to practice other ways of taking care of your temptations and emotional needs. That's one of the reasons Amy stresses the importance of figuring out alternate ways of soothing yourself and meeting whatever needs exist. A lot of people struggle more at night or when they first get home from work because they feel like they deserve a reward for getting through the day and their reward used to be food. That means that you need to come up with other physical pleasures you can have instead of food, like a massage, sex, soaking in a warm bath, or some other kind of "feel-good" reward. Since food gives you physical satisfaction and releases endorphins, it's important that you find other activities that will also give you a sense of physical satisfaction and create good feelings.

When I told a friend about trading the food addiction for the shopping addiction she suggested that I make a game of *not* buying, just like I make up games to keep from overeating. She said, "When I go into a store, my game is to see if I can leave without buying anything at all." I immediately blurted out, "I'm not playing that game! I'm not ready for that." We both laughed, because we knew it was true. A few weeks ago one of the shopping channels was making a garden hose sound so amazing that I caught myself reaching for my credit card. Then I suddenly realized, "Hey, I don't have a garden!" To keep winning, you've got to be more honest with yourself than you've ever been before. If you're not, you will sabotage your own efforts by trying to do things that you're not yet ready or able to do.

Recruit Your Winning Team

Amy says, "When you're heavy, it's easy to attribute many of your problems to your weight. Once you lose the weight, all the skill deficits that you didn't know you had because you were avoiding things get uncovered. Since society is structured to revere being thin and losing weight, you really are set up to be taken by surprise when you realize how hard it is to live even when you're thin." When that reality sets in, people tend to blame themselves and put themselves down for having a difficult time dealing with things. Amy says, "In order to really forgive yourself for all those struggles, you have to realize that you are trying to learn how to handle things that other people have had decades to learn how to manage. And you're learning all these things without using what used to be your most reliable source of comfort—overeating. So you are very strong and brave! Try to keep in mind that you can't learn everything at once and that criticizing yourself slows down the learning process and just makes everything that much more difficult."

This is when it's really important to find other people who are in the same boat as you are, and also to be proactive by inviting people you admire and trust to be part of your maintenance support team.

You probably have some friends and family members who think that now that you've lost weight, you should be happy every day of your life. I hear this all the time. Some of my friends tell me I no longer have any reason to be unhappy.

I called my girlfriend Teena recently to reach out and tell her I was down and she said, "Why are you down? You are writing a book!" God, I wish it were that simple.

These people, though you may love them very much, are not the ones you want on your support team! Instead, recruit a small group of people who understand that your problems didn't disappear with your excess pounds and that keeping those pounds off forever is going to require your complete commitment, strength, perseverance, and their support. Share your goals and your game plan with them and let them know how important they will be to your success.

TWENTY-FIVE YEARS AND GOING STRONG!

One of the women that I'm really inspired by is Florence Tannen, a friend of my mother's who lost ninety pounds when she was in her forties and has kept it off for more than twenty-five years. Florence was a size 9 when she got married, gained weight during her first pregnancy, gained more weight during her second pregnancy, and just kept gaining until she reached 225 pounds. She said, "I was disgusted with myself, but I couldn't get it together and stop eating. Life itself overwhelmed me. When I finally decided to go to OA (Overeaters Anonymous) and then to therapy, I found out that I had never learned the basic skills that I needed to get through a day without turning to food. I had no discipline and very little motivation. I cared, but I didn't care. When I learned that over-eating was a symptom of other problems that I had rather than the problem itself, I was astonished. When I discovered that under my nice, smiling, accommodating personality, I was not only angry, but also enraged, I was shocked. Who me, angry? I really couldn't believe it at first. How could I have gone all those years without knowing I was so angry?"

Florence committed to turning her pain into power and over the years won back her self-respect and the respect of others. She said, "I love food and food is always going to be a part of my life, so I don't want to think of it as the enemy. People with drug or alcohol addictions have the option of taking that substance out of their life entirely and in some ways the all-or-nothing approach seems like it would be easier. We can't do that with food. We have to eat to live, and if we never allow ourselves to have something that tastes good, we're going to feel too deprived and probably end up bingeing or gaining again. I still struggle sometimes, but for the most part I've learned to wrap my arms around food and embrace it like a friend. I eat very healthy foods most of the time and think they taste great."

She said that when she finds herself overindulging again or realizes that she's put on a few pounds, those are cues that tell her it's time to regroup. She said, "When I realize I'm off track I get back on. I don't say,

'Oh well, too late now. I might as well eat a pint of ice cream.' That would be like breaking an arm and saying, 'Oh well, I broke my arm, I might as well break my other arm and maybe a leg or two.'"

Every single person who has kept the weight off understands and lives by what Florence just said. They don't let one misstep lead to another. If they blow it, they pick themselves up and start all over again.

Florence explained, "A few months ago I knew I needed support again, so I went to OA and got back in touch with the practices that work for me. I can't tell people that someday their struggle will be over, but I can tell them that the more they practice living and eating with moderation, the better at it they will get and the less they will have to constantly think about it."

The Florences of the world let us know that yes, it sure is possible, and we *can* do it!

Cope with Your Regrets

There is nothing you can do to change your past. But there are a lot of things you can do to change your life today and in all the days to come. You have to accept the past—the things you did and the things you didn't get to do. To do that, you need to train yourself to turn your mind away from regrets and toward possibilities. When you catch yourself obsessing over your regrets, imagine yourself turning the page, as if your life is a book and you're flipping to a new page, which represents today. Then take a look around you and notice how many choices you have. Switch your focus from negative to positive. Think about all the new and exciting changes in your life.

Amy says, "Changing your thinking from regrets to gratitude is not an overnight process; so don't expect miracles when you first start doing this. The important thing is identifying and recognizing the negative thoughts and willing yourself to replace them with something more realistic and positive. Sometimes you'll only have a few moments of acceptance or peace before your mind goes back to the regret or negative thought. That's normal. If you've been thinking or saying negative things to yourself hundreds of times a day for years, it will take saying positive things to yourself hundreds of times a day for years for your new way of thinking to become second nature. So don't get discouraged or give up if you don't feel a difference after only a few days or weeks. Just like it took time for you to shed the pounds, it will take time for you to shed the old negative ways of thinking and distance yourself from your regrets."

When You Can't Think Positively, Distract Yourself!

There will also be times when trying to turn your mind toward positive thoughts just doesn't work. When that happens, you have to distract yourself by doing something that forces you to concentrate. You might read, file paperwork, balance your checkbook, or organize a closet or some drawers. Experiment and find out what activities occupy your mind in a way that you can't simultaneously be thinking about negative things or fretting over something that is beyond your control. For me, cleaning kills three birds with one stone. I get more organized, it burns calories, and it takes my mind off my negative thoughts.

Howard, a member of the Winners' Circle for seven years, says he collects one-minute mystery books and uses them to force him to think of something besides his problems. "I've gotten good at turning my attention from the things I can't control to things I can do something about, but once in a while something will still get me and twist me around like a flag flapping in the wind. If I can't let it go after half an hour, I pull out one of my one-minute mystery books and work on one of the cases I haven't solved yet. I read the story and then go about my business. My goal is to solve the mystery in twenty-four hours. When I do it, I treat myself to a ten-minute chair massage at my office building. If I don't solve it in twenty-four hours, I still win because it keeps my mind occupied until I figure it out. And by that time, whatever had me worked up doesn't seem so important."

HOT TIP
The Dish on Plates

When you eat out, ask your server to bring you a take-home box when he or she brings your meal.

Immediately divide the meal into two portions by putting half of it in the box. Think of it as a twofer—two for the price of one. And you know we don't need Flintstone portions anyway. (Remember at the beginning of each episode when the ribs at the drive-thru tip over Fred's car?) Yabba-dabba-doo!

Accept the Things You Cannot Change

When you first start thinking about the things you can't change, you may not always be realistic. There will probably be things you feel you should be able to change that you can't, and things you think you have to live with that you can actually change.

Turning pain into power includes making peace with the things you honestly cannot change. If you continue to harbor grief, regret, and disappointment over these things, you can lose sight of all the positive changes that you *have* made and *can* make to improve your life now and in the future.

Take out your Winners' Circle Workbook and make two lists. Call the first list "Things I Want to Change/Improve" and write everything that you want to change on this list. Call the second list "Things I Want to Learn to Accept" and on this list write down all the things you wish you could change, but know or believe that you can't. Working with a life coach or therapist on these lists can make a world of difference, but if you're not ready or willing to do that, just seeing the items on each list can help you to start sorting out how you're feeling. It can also help you decide what you want to work on. You can't do everything at once, so choose just one or two things from each list at a time. Pick the two highest-priority changes that you want to make and the top one or two things you want to learn to accept, and work on those until you feel okay about them. Then pick one or two more things from each of your lists.

You'll notice that the items on your lists will change as you progress and grow. Some of the goals on your "Want to Change" list will become less important and you might decide you don't want to change some of them after all. Some of the things on your "Learn to Accept" list will be resolved or you won't regret them anymore.

For example, Joanne, a member of the Winners' Circle, had written on her "Learn to Accept" list that she never had children and now she is too old to have them. She said when she got married, she and her husband agreed they'd start a family in a few years, and they even had a room they called the nursery in the house they built. But three years turned into five, and in the meantime, Joanne was working a desk job and going to school for her master's degree, and before she knew it, she'd gained fifteen pounds. That year on the couple's anniversary she asked her husband when they could start their family. She said, "He looked at me with disgust and said, 'When you lose weight. If you get pregnant now you'll break the bed.' That was the beginning of the end of my marriage, although I didn't want to admit it then. It was a long, ugly divorce and by the time it was final, my fertile years were all but over. I thought about artificial insemination and considered adopting, but I didn't want to be a single parent. For several years, I couldn't get over my anger and disappointment at missing out on having kids. Then last year I got the job of my dreams. I get to travel all over the world and I love it! The thing is that I'm away more than I'm home and there's no way I could have accepted this job if I was raising a family. I'm not saying a job is more important than a family, but for where I am in my life, I can now see that I'm much happier with my freedom and getting to see the world than I'd be if I were at home changing diapers."

Some common issues on "Learn to Accept" lists include:

1. The Number of Years You've Lost

This is a biggie because you can't turn back time and you can't really make up for lost time either. What you *can* do is discover what you gained during the time you think you lost. For instance, I discovered I love to write and I love public speaking and I sharpened my people skills and I am very intuitive about life. I discovered a sense of humor as a way to survive. If I had the choice, I probably wouldn't decide to do it again, but being overweight has taught me a lot. It has made me very kind and it has made me attracted to kind people.

The other important point here is that every minute that you dwell on what you think you've lost is another minute you lose from your present life. I don't know about you, but I don't want to give up even a millisecond more!

2. The Toll That Being Overweight Has Taken on
    Your Body

Even though you can't reverse all the damage you did to
your body, you can take the best possible care of yourself
from this day forward. In fact, you now have a chance to be
the healthiest and most fit that you've ever been. By exercising, eating right, and taking care of your mental health, you
can enjoy a quality of life that many people—even those
who are thin—never experience. Some people also choose
to have reconstructive surgery to improve their mobility,
health, and the way they look. (To make an informed decision about plastic surgery, read the sidebar in this chapter
on what plastic surgery can and can't do.)

Sometimes You Have to Say Good-Bye

Hard as it can be, sometimes you have to be willing to end a
relationship that you know isn't good for you. You also have
to be able to deal with it when other people choose to end a
relationship with you. There will be certain people who will
never let themselves see the new you, and there might be
a few you need to move on from. Please don't fret. It hurts
at the time, but when one door closes another one opens.
I promise. The hurt will lessen. One of my best friends in
the world walked away from me when he saw I was finally
okay. He was around to see the dramatic weight changes
but he never got to see the dramatic life changes afterward.
I wish he was with me to enjoy all the new activities I can

now do. In the past, all we really did was eat and hang out at my apartment. Once in a while the sadness comes up about this, but then I let it go and I focus on all the new people in my life and all the new playgrounds I have and the new playmates that I see every day.

Just about everyone in the Winners' Circle has a story or two to tell about a friendship, intimate relationship, or family tie that was severed while they were losing weight or shortly after they reached their goal weight.

Jocelyn, who has successfully kept the weight off for three years, said the hardest thing she ever did was leave her fiancé, who was an alcoholic. She said, "When I was overeating and he was drinking every night, somehow it worked. But when I started losing weight and wasn't numbing out with food anymore, I started to see how empty our relationship was, and I sort of became like his mother. I went from being his partner in crime to scolding him and being annoyed when he forgot to pick up the dry cleaning. I got pissed off that I bothered to make a nice dinner when he was barely sober enough to eat it and passed out without bothering to help clean up first." She said what shocked her though was that for months she was convinced that his drinking had gotten worse and that's why he was so hard to put up with. "One day," she said, "I was on the phone with my sister complaining about him and she said, 'Nick's been like that for as long as I've known him.' My sister knew him longer than I did. We all lived in the same town. When she said that, my mind did this fast rewind back through the five years we lived together and I realized my sister was right. I could hardly believe that I went for years without noticing that stuff, or without noticing it enough for it to bother me. It's been a year since I left him. I guess I still love him in some ways, but I know I did the right thing."

Liz, who has maintained her goal weight for four years, said that when her older sister came to visit and saw her as a size 10 for the first time, their closeness came to a screeching halt. Liz said, "I still don't understand what happened. We were close our whole lives. Some people said she was jealous, but she was always the beauty in the family and was never overweight, so I can't imagine what she would have been jealous about. But when she came to visit, as soon as she saw me, she started to act weird. She lives in another state so I hadn't seen her in over two years, but the whole time I was losing weight, we talked on the phone every week and she encouraged me to keep it up and sent me fat-free snacks and funny cards to make me feel good. But then when she was here, she accused me of having liposuction and said I couldn't have gone from a 14 to a 10 just by being on a diet and exercising. The whole thing was really crazy and it still hurts. When I call her now, she's polite, but distant. It's like she's a whole different person. I'm glad I lost weight, but I wish I didn't have to lose my sister with it."

Amy explains, "Whenever people make progress, they also experience loss, and that loss can come in many different forms. Most people want to believe that moving forward—making progress—is all positive and they want to do it without experiencing anything painful. So one of the most important parts of turning pain into power is accepting that moving forward means leaving certain behaviors and sometimes even people behind. You can't hold on to the past and grab on to the future at the same time." Trying to do that will literally pull you apart.

Renewing Good Relationships and Re-creating Not-So-Good Ones

If there are family members and friends that you lost touch with because you were too embarrassed to see them when you were heavy, you can probably renew some of those relationships if you're willing to humble yourself and be honest with them about what you've been going through. Before I lost weight, I spent a lot of time alone because I didn't feel good enough about myself to let people into my life. But over the past few years I've learned that the people who love me have loved me all along, whether I was fat or not.

My mother is my biggest fan and greatest supporter and always has been, but there were many times that I shut her out of my life too. She's always wanted what was best for me and couldn't understand why I kept her at a distance. She cried when she told me there were years when she felt like she had lost her daughter. At the time, I was in too much of my own pain to understand the pain that I was causing her and my other family members.

My brother Mal used to get so upset when I wouldn't attend family functions or let him visit me when he came to town. He was concerned about my health, but he was never upset by my weight. Renewing my relationship with him is one of the best things that I've done! So if there are people you want to invite back into your life, now is the time to do it. Just be prepared that some people will have moved on and might feel like there's been too much water under the bridge to pick up where you left off. But most people will be happy to be back in your life.

Chances are there are also some relationships that you don't consider healthy or supportive, but you still want to maintain them or re-create them because they are with people you can't or are not willing to eliminate from your life. For example, Toya, a member of the Winners' Circle for three years, said she never got along with her brother-in-law, Bobby, but she loves her sister and her nieces and nephews, so she was constantly trying to find a way to smooth the waves with him.

She said, "I tried everything I could think of, but every time I was at their house, he managed to say something rude or condescending to me. I gave their family gifts every year at Christmas and he never once thanked me. He just acted like I didn't get him anything and my sister thanked me for him. After I lost weight, it got worse. He started to taunt me with food. At first I thought I was paranoid, but when other people started to notice it, I knew he was trying to tempt me. I'd show up to visit and he'd go out and come back a half hour later with cakes, cookies, and gallons of ice cream. I was so upset because I really thought for a while that I might have to stop going over there, and the idea of not seeing my sister and the kids practically broke my heart. Thank goodness I told the minister at my church about it, because she gave me a way to handle it that's working.

"She told me that in some Native American tribes they call people like Bobby a good enemy. She said to think of him as a teacher who is helping me to increase my willpower, strength, and commitment. She also said that a good enemy can give us a chance to learn to accept and be more compassionate with people we don't like. She said, 'It's easy to love and be nice to people that you like and approve of, but if you can learn to love Bobby, honey, your soul will grow by leaps and bounds!'"

A Dozen Paths to Empowerment

Wishes get you nothing, decisions get you everything.

1.   Clarify What's Most Important to You

Dr. Nadler says to imagine that you are the only person in the entire world whom you have to please and to figure out what you would most love to do with your life. Ask yourself, "What does success mean to me? What do I most want to accomplish before I die?"

She says, "This may sound morbid, but sit down and write your own obituary. Write it as if you lived to be at least ninety-five and you are describing everything that you did with your life that you feel proud of and good about. Doing that will help you to get to the heart of what's most important to you."

2. Exchange Fantasy for Possibility

Self-empowerment relies on being willing to exchange your fantasies for possibilities. Dr. Nadler says, "I'm not saying that you should limit yourself or go after less than what you want in life. Just make sure that what you want is truly possible and achievable in some form."

3. Be Responsible for Your Own Happiness

Dr. Nadler says the path to self-empowerment is paved with your own choices and actions. She says, "Accept that you are responsible for your own happiness. Stop waiting for someone else to entertain you, approve of you, rescue you, or fall in love with you. It's nice when those things happen, but learn how to make your own happiness so you're not reliant on what other people choose to do or not do."

4. Quit Playing the Blame Game

"Ultimately, I've never seen blame lead to a win, either for the person doing the blaming or the person being blamed," explains Dr. Nadler. She says, "If you want to succeed at winning after losing, you've got to give up the anger and the blame."

5. Laugh

Laughter and humor are lifesavers. Very few things can turn pain into power as well as laughing until you have tears in your eyes.

Dr. Nadler says, "If you're really serious all the time you'll feel heavy, even if you only weigh a hundred pounds. Plus, laughter has proven health benefits, so treat yourself to a good laugh!" (Personally, laughter has been my savior many, many times!)

6.   Appreciate the Beauty That Surrounds You

Dr. Nadler says, "Sometimes all it takes is one colorful flower or the radiant smile of a child to lift your mood and make you feel good. Beauty is all around us, and most of it is free—watching a sunrise or a sunset, taking in the beauty of a garden that you pass on your way to work, or stopping to admire a painting in the hall outside your office. Appreciate the beauty that surrounds you and find ways to bring more beauty into your life."

7.   Stay Connected

Amy says, "Plan to spend time with the people you love and the people who you know are good influences on you. When you feel depressed or you find yourself withdrawing and are tempted to isolate yourself, reach out to someone instead. There is a lot to be said about time spent alone, but most people find alone time more enjoyable when they're feeling good about themselves."

8.   Be Active

You don't have to be a gym bunny to be active, and being active doesn't always have to mean exercising. Amy says,

"Being physically active is transforming. Our bodies evolved to be physically active, so we feel best when we're doing something with them. You can walk, run, skip rope, swim, dance, do yoga, garden, or clean your house. The idea is simply to move instead of staying still."

9. Be Proactive About Your Emotional Needs

Stay in touch with yourself and be honest about the struggles that can make you want to numb out with food so you can plan how you're going to win those battles ahead of time. For example, Amy says, "If something happens that upsets you emotionally, assess the situation and your state of mind and decide what you need. If you know you can get through the day but you're concerned about the evening, pick up the phone and make plans to spend the evening with a friend, assign yourself a project to do, or plan to go to a movie or do something that will give your mind a mini-vacation. Think of it like putting up a net before you walk across the tightrope."

10. Know That Your Opinion of Yourself Matters Most

Frequently remind yourself that what you think of yourself matters more than what anyone else thinks of you. Amy says, "If you've struggled with feeling good about yourself, it's easy to believe the negative things that other people say about you, but that doesn't mean those things are true. A lot of times the criticisms that people make about others have more to do with themselves than with the person they're criticizing. Remember that when someone says, 'Do you want to know what I think?' or some form of that, you have every right to say, 'No thank you.'"

11.   Give Therapy a Fair Chance

Finding the right person to help you can be life-altering. You should know after three or four sessions if the therapist you're seeing is right for you. If it's not right, try someone else. But make sure you're trying a new therapist because you're looking for the right fit, not because you're trying to avoid feeling uncomfortable. Amy says, "You can expect to feel uncomfortable from time to time, but you can also expect to have a therapist who really understands what you're experiencing and can help you to make sense of it. It's not always about having huge 'Aha' moments. It's great when that happens, but it's just as valuable to learn to accept yourself and learn how to cope with and manage the people and issues in your life that are challenging."

12.   Be Gentle with Yourself

Amy says, "Practice treating yourself like a cherished friend— in your thoughts and your actions. Focus on what you like about yourself and cut yourself slack in the areas where you know you have room for improvement. Give yourself the credit you deserve and share your accomplishments with the people you love and care about. Make time to celebrate your progress and the achievement of your goals."

Getting Naked

People who have lost weight tend to see their bodies differently than how they really look. Even people who were never heavy can be very critical of their appearance. (Even supermodels are airbrushed!) A lot of people look in the mirror and say horrible things that they would never even dream of saying to their worst enemies. Amy says, "Some people have a condition that's called body dysmorphic disorder. When you have this condition, you think your small imperfections are major disfigurements." For example, if you have a little bit of a belly, you think you look nine months pregnant. Another example is an average-size woman who thinks of herself as huge. The important thing is to discover the truth of how you really appear in the mirror versus what is in your eyes only.

Amy explains, "Your body image is based on two things: how your body looks and how it works. Sometimes people get so preoccupied with how they look that they forget or downplay how strong and able their bodies are. People who don't like the way their bodies look or who feel embarrassed about them decide that they can't go swimming in public, or they can't go to the gym or wear shorts. This way of thinking frequently leads to, 'I don't like my body, so I can't have sex.'" So try really hard to separate how your body looks from how it works because doing that will build more confidence and help you to feel more freedom about what you are able and willing to do. "By using your body and having physically enjoyable experiences you can improve how you feel and how you look." That's an important and valuable step toward increasing your own comfort level!

Basically, before you can feel more comfortable being naked in front of someone else, you have to get more comfortable with the way you see yourself. You can work toward this by doing a desensitization exercise. This exercise is challenging, but it works for a lot of people, so I hope you'll try it.

Desensitization Exercise

Read all of the instruction before you begin. Amy recommends that you practice this exercise twice a week until you can look at yourself and feel okay about what you see.

Take off your clothes and stand in front of a full-length mirror. Breathe slowly and deeply and try to think of the person in the mirror as a good friend, someone you want to be kind to and don't want to hurt or criticize. Practice being objective as you look at the image in front of you. Say gentle, neutral things about what you observe. For example, instead of saying, "Those are huge saddlebags," try saying, "My thighs are curved there."

Amy says, "When you're looking in the mirror, you should stay there for at least ten or fifteen minutes. The important thing is to stay in front of the mirror until you are no longer feeling intense anxiety. If you quit in the middle of the intense anxiety, then you're reinforcing the escape, which isn't helpful. You want your mind and body to start to calm down so you can start having neutral sensations that go along with the neutral things you're saying to yourself." That really is important, because if you only look at yourself for five minutes and don't stay there long enough to start seeing yourself at least a little more objectively, you can feel worse instead of better, put on your clothes, and head right for the kitchen. Don't go there!

She says, "By describing your body in more neutral ways, you can train yourself to be less judgmental of yourself, which can open the door for you to go to the gym or the pool more regularly, and that will in turn help you to release endorphins and improve your self-esteem, not to mention your muscle tone." The more you use your body, the more pleasure you will feel and the better you will feel about yourself. The better you feel about yourself, the better you can feel when you're with your partner or a lover. Now, this is something worth working on! How are you supposed to achieve orgasm if you're thinking about the cellulite in your thighs? Your sexual pleasure, just like everything else in your life, begins with you. As Amy and many other wise women have pointed out, when you feel sexy, you *are* sexy. People get turned on by your energy and your personality. It's more about how you feel and how your partner feels than about how either of you look. Still, there's a lot to be said about pretty nightgowns, darkness, or very, very soft candlelight!

I asked the first few guys I dated if it would be all right with them if I pleased them, without them doing anything to satisfy me. They were totally bewildered because they had no idea that keeping my clothes on was my way of hiding my low self-esteem. Now I know that my low self-esteem was not so much under my clothes as it was between my ears.

When my relationship with my first boyfriend got intimate, I refused to take off my clothes because even at night it was too bright in my apartment because of all the city lights outside my window. I told my boyfriend that if he wanted to have sex, he'd have to put up blinds. The next day he showed up with a toolbox, a drill, blinds, and all the hardware to hang them. He got rewarded!

I would like to think that someday I'll be able to take my clothes off in front of a man without being afraid of rejection, but I know it will take someone very special. Years ago I saw a movie about a woman who was a burn victim. Her entire body, except for her face, was covered with scars. I don't remember the name of the movie, but the memory stuck with me because of the way the leading man was able to accept and love her. During one of the movie's last scenes, they are about to make love and she pulls her arms up to try and cover her body. He gently moves her arms and looks at her with complete love and adoration in his eyes as he says, "You're beautiful the way you are." When it comes to the acceptance that most women are hoping for, that scene says it all.

WHAT PLASTIC SURGERY CAN AND CAN'T DO

One of the most common complaints of people who have lost a significant amount of weight is loose or hanging skin. Some people think of this as an "appearance" issue only, but if you have a great deal of extra skin it can cause problems with your health and your mobility. There are two basic categories of plastic surgery: cosmetic and reconstructive. Dr. Andrew Elkwood explains, "The purpose of cosmetic surgery is to take something that is 'normal' and improve or enhance it. Reconstructive surgery takes something that is a problem and fixes it so that it is normal or as close to normal as possible. If you're thinking about having surgery, you need to educate yourself about the procedure you're considering, choose a qualified surgeon that you trust, and make sure you understand the limitations of the procedure and the possible complications."

Dr. Elkwood says, "Plastic surgery is not magic. It can be transforming and give you a psychological boost, but it should be an answer to a specific anatomic problem. It shouldn't be an answer to the woes of life. It can't save your marriage, make your boyfriend or girlfriend respect you, or make you a better person. If you had no self-esteem before, you'll have no self-esteem after. One of the most important things you can do for yourself if you're considering surgery is to make sure you have realistic expectations. If you don't, you shouldn't seek surgery and no one should perform surgery."

One of the things you need to know is that you will have scars and there's no way to tell how noticeable or unattractive the scar is going to be until after you heal from the surgery. So it's important to decide which is the lesser of evils for you, the hanging skin or the scars. For me, the "beauty" scars won hands down. Not just because I couldn't stand the way the hanging skin looked, but because it was having a serious, negative effect on my health and my mobility.

Dr. Elkwood says, "Whenever you have surgery there is always the possibility of complications. Some of the complications include asymmetry, need for further surgery, need to touch something up, disfigurement, numbness, pain, excess bleeding and need for a blood transfusion, and risk of infection and death. It's real surgery and should be taken very seriously. It's not la-di-da. If a surgeon tells you that there is no risk of complications or that they've never had a patient with complications, run."

To select a surgeon, first confirm that he or she is certified with the American Board of Plastic Surgery. Get references from your own doctor and from other people who have had the same surgery that you're considering. Make sure the surgeon you choose has performed the procedure you're seeking many, many times and that he or she is willing and able to thoroughly answer all of your questions. Dr. Elkwood says, "You also should ask to see before-and-after photos, not so much to see the quality of their work, because they're always going to show you their best photos, but because you want to make sure they can piece together a large enough portfolio of the type of surgery you're considering."

He says, "If a surgeon is telling you that he does something that no one else does, the procedure he's doing is probably not very good. Every once in a while there needs to be a first person or a second person before the hundredth person doing something, but that's few and far between. The cosmetic surgery market is so competitive that there are few worthwhile things for cosmetic purposes that one person is doing that the others are not. Most of the time, it pans out to be a marketing thing."

Dr. Elkwood says, "Unfortunately there are a lot of snake-oil salesmen and predators out there. Most of the time slippery people are better at presenting themselves than upstanding people because they survive on showmanship. So you need to be very careful. Use common sense, use your gut, and remember that if it sounds too good to be true, it usually is. For example, a surgeon who charges a higher price isn't necessarily better than someone charging less, but if a surgeon is offering a lower-than-average price, that's probably a sign that she's not very busy. I have this saying: 'Don't buy discount sushi and don't buy discount surgery.' I'm happy to pay full price for my sushi."

Crank Up Your Sexual Joy Meter

One of the best things about growing emotionally and increasing your self-esteem is that you start to believe that you deserve to have your own needs and desires met! In the bedroom (or wherever you are!), knowing that you deserve to feel good is a critical part of really enjoying yourself. And don't forget, you *do* deserve to enjoy yourself! One of your partner's greatest pleasures will be seeing your enjoyment. As well it should be!

Sexual satisfaction has a lot to do with how well you understand your body, and knowing what you like, what works for you and what doesn't. That's why it's so important and fun to do some exploring. (Ponce de Leon had nothing on me!) You can find out a lot about yourself, and that will keep you from getting stuck in a rut. So set out on a voyage of sexual self-discovery. Ahoy, matey!

It's natural for people who have recently lost weight to be a little out of touch with their own bodies. (I'd ignored mine for so many years that it just seemed natural to only focus from the chin up.) So the first step to cranking up your sexual joy meter is to go back to Sex Class 101 by touching yourself in a variety of ways (yee-ha!), using different motions and different amounts of pressure. Figure out what turns you on and where you are most sensitive. Does it feel better when you're lying on your side or your back? Are you more excited if your legs are up or down, wide open or close together? If you want to expand your repertoire, buy a book or video that can give you more information about your body and some new ideas and different techniques that can spice up your sex life. Talk to your chatty friends who just love to gossip about this stuff. To turn up the heat even more, buy a sex toy. Learn how you like to use the toy, and if you have a partner, find out how you can use it with him or her. I have to admit that one of my favorite things to do is to go into a shop where they sell the toys and ask lots of questions. The people who work in those shops are trained to keep a straight face and answer questions as comfortably as if you just asked, "Do you sell tubs of butter?" instead of "Can I get the lubricant in a gallon-size drum?"

Creating the Sexual Connection You Crave

Dr. Greer says, "Another benefit of becoming more emotionally aware and secure is being willing to take some small risks and putting yourself out there a little to create the sexual connection that you crave. The first step is to learn how to balance the give-and-take and make sure that both your and your partner's needs and desires are being fed equally. Since everyone has different tastes, preferences, and sex drives, one of the biggest hurdles is being willing to stretch your boundaries and learn to appreciate some of each other's favorites. In those cases where you and your partner are really at odds, this can be a little like trying to enjoy a food that turns your stomach, but with some creativity, it can be done! One way to increase your tolerance level for an activity you're not crazy about, or really don't like, is to focus on how much pleasure your partner derives from it. For example, if you'd rather scrub the floor than give your mate oral sex, take as much of your attention off of yourself as you can and really try to get into his or her level of excitement and the pleasure that you are providing for someone you love. You can also work toward increasing your appreciation for a particular activity the same way you might cultivate a taste for a food that's good for you, but that you don't like. For instance, if oral sex is not your cup of tea, instead of feeling that you have to take his entire penis in your mouth, you can just lick the shaft or swirl your tongue around the tip while you stroke him with your hand. Get some flavored edible massage oil and pretend you're eating a lollipop. The idea is to keep trying different variations on a sexual theme until you find a couple that are palatable."

It's also very important to find at least a handful of activities that you both really enjoy. Think of these as your entrees and include each other's favorites as appetizers, side dishes, and desserts—even if you're only up for a few bites. (I still compare everything to food. Did you ever ask a fat person for directions? They'll say something like this: "Make a left at the Dunkin' Donuts, go three stoplights, and turn at the Burger King.")

Dr. Greer says, "Another important part of creating the connection you desire is being willing to take turns being responsible for setting the mood and the theme for the evening. If you are a romantic and your most satisfying sex involves candlelight, soft music, and flowers, encourage your partner to try and create this scenario for you. If your mate is into extreme passion, complete with let's-get-it-on quickie sex, then go along with it and occasionally thrill him with the unexpected by initiating that kind of sex yourself. By being willing to go the distance for each other, as well as meeting each other halfway, you can both feast on your sexual connection and feed your closeness and trust at the same time."

THE IMPERFECT TEN

The Top Ten Reasons to Turn Your Emotional Pain into Power

1. Because you deserve it!
2. Even though anger sometimes feels like a comfortable old shoe and makes you feel justified, letting go of it will feel like the best thing you've ever experienced.
3. It will set you free!
4. Emotional suffering consumes way too much of your time, which can be spent on much better things.
5. Your emotional well-being is directly related to your ability to *maintain* your weight!
6. You don't want to feel physically drained all the time—turning your pain into power will give you more energy.

7. Letting go of the painful part of your past allows you to embrace the present and future.

8. It will make it easier to help the loved ones in your life whom you just can't figure out how to help. Being a good example of leading a positive lifestyle is the most powerful way to help someone else.

9. Holding on to pain leads to a possible gain (on the scale).

10. POWER = CHOICE!

STEP 4

Appreciate Small Victories
The Little Things Are Everything

Anyone who keeps the ability to see
Beauty never grows old.

—Franz Kafka, *Saturday Review*

Appreciating every small step you take in the right direction and all the little things that life has to offer are two of the smartest things you can do. I've been doing this for so long now that it just sounds like common sense, but having common sense and using it are two different things. A lot of people think that if they don't climb a mountain, or do something else just as big, they're not making progress or that the progress they did make wasn't worth much. But making progress isn't about climbing mountains; it's about walking over one molehill after another. Eventually you'll have taken so many small steps that they'll add up to a mountain's worth. If there's one thing I know for sure, it's that maintaining your weight isn't about the mountains, it's about the molehills.

Step 4 in *Winning After Losing* is about shifting your attention from negative to positive by celebrating your victories—instead of kvetching about your problems or wallowing in your defeats. It's about appreciating the small pleasures in life that many people overlook or take for granted. The little things really do have the power to change your life and make you the happiest. The trick is to acknowledge and celebrate your small victories and to slow down enough to enjoy life's simple pleasures. In this chapter, you'll learn how to keep track of your victories, build your emotional muscles, celebrate your accomplishments, get really real with yourself, increase your comfort, confidence, and self-respect, and savor the joy of simple pleasures.

Document and Share Your Victories

People usually think of victories as really big things, but if you do that, you cheat yourself out of feeling good about all the things you accomplish every day. Members of the Winners' Circle know that keeping a list of their small victories and sharing their "wins" with their family and friends helps them to stay motivated. It also keeps them from disregarding small steps and simple kindnesses that add up to major personal growth and progress. Just saying no to the second doughnut is a victory! Trying new things, going new places, making new friends, dating, or reigniting the romance in your relationship are all worth celebrating. But if you don't make it a habit to acknowledge yourself for these things, it's

easy to overlook them and feel like you're not accomplishing much of anything. By keeping track of your molehills, your firsts, and every small victory that you have, you begin to realize that the little things are everything and your daily life becomes happier, more meaningful, and more fun. Trust me!

Record Your Small Victories

Create a special section in your Winners' Circle Workbook to keep track of every small victory. Each time you do something that is proof of your new way of living, make a note of it in your "Small Victories" section. If you don't carry your workbook with you, then note these victories on a piece of paper, Post-it notes, or in your Palm Pilot so you can transfer them to your workbook at the end of each day. Don't let more than one day go by before you write them down because then you'll be tempted to disregard some of the smaller ones—or forget them—and only record the ones that you think are more impressive. And that defeats the point of the exercise! The funny thing is that the molehills have always been my mountains—something like red being the new black this season. (The small victories have always been the first things I tell people about when they ask how my life has changed. If being able to tie your own shoes without pain isn't a mountain, I don't know what is!) The reason you should keep track of each and every thing, no matter how small it might seem (for at least a few months),

is to train your mind to notice and pay attention to all the small but significant things you accomplish every day. If you don't add at least four or five items to your Small Victories list each day, you're probably not giving yourself enough credit.

Sample of One Day's Small Victories

Walked up two flights of stairs instead of taking the elevator.

Didn't eat one of the doughnuts that coworker brought in to work.

Took a five-minute walk around the block after lunch instead of having a cup of coffee.

Made a phone call that I didn't want to make and had been avoiding.

Ate my afternoon snack (an apple) in the lunchroom, instead of at my desk.

Looked in the mirror and complimented myself on my smile and the way my pants fit.

Another important part of celebrating small victories is sharing them with other people. Don't keep all that joy and excitement to yourself! The people who care about you want to know about the good things you're experiencing. Plus, sharing your accomplishments with other people can help you to appreciate them more yourself. Don't let a single day go by without taking notice and appreciating how you and your life have improved.

ENJOYING WHAT YOU USED TO DREAD

There are countless small victories to celebrate in this category alone, and when you add them all up, they definitely make a mountain of molehills! You'll have your own stack of molehills, but I'm guessing that many people who have lost weight will be able to relate to some of the same things. For example, a lot of those who only have ten or fifteen pounds to lose dread summer and warm weather. Personally, the sound of lawn mowers in the spring always used to make me shudder because I knew that within weeks I'd have to emerge from all the layers of clothing I wore in the winter. I also hated that summer days had so many hours of light and used to wish the hours would speed by so I could be covered by the dark of night. I thought of nighttime as an accessory because I was convinced it made me look thinner! Summer is also the season for wicker furniture. Need I say more?

Selections from the Winners' Circle

Loveseats! Being able to comfortably fit on one with another person.
Wearing shorts. (No more thigh chafing!)
Sleeveless shirts. (Gone are the upper-arm "wings"!)
Shopping for new clothes.
Class reunions.
Sexual encounters.
Scales and the nurse in the doctor's office who smiles as she says, "Please step up."

Booths at restaurants. (Knowing I can now fit in them!)
Dropping my pen (or anything else).
Shoes with laces.
Getting on crowded elevators without fear of exceeding
    the maximum load.

Building Your Emotional Muscles
Takes Time and Practice

If you want to appreciate your small victories but they seem insignificant compared with the challenges you face every day, keep in mind that when you're making progress in your life, you're usually going uphill. As we've said, you may have thought that losing weight was going to be the steepest part of the climb, but now that you're in the maintenance stage, you know that keeping the weight off is even harder. So until your new way of living becomes as natural as brushing your teeth every day, you are walking uphill. As Amy says, "When you first start up the hill, you're not in shape yet, so the first year or so is going to be more painful and difficult and may make you wonder what in the world you have to appreciate or celebrate—especially when problems come up that you never had to face before!" At times like those (and we all have them!), life may seem worse instead of better. But people who have maintained their goal weight for more than a few years can assure you that if you keep at this until it truly becomes a way of life, it does get easier and it is definitely worth it! Applauding yourself for the small things will help you make it to the five-year marker, and then the ten-year and beyond!

Remember that every new thing you try takes learning and practice. And remember, too, that no matter how much practice you get, you are not going to be perfect. No one is perfect. (It's about progress, not perfection.) The beauty is that you can and will get better and better! For instance, if you only spent one day doing yoga, you'd probably spend the rest of your life wondering what in the hell other people like about it. You'd be tired, sore, and possibly miserable. But if you did it a few days a week for a month, gradually learning one position after another, your muscles would get stronger and become more flexible and toned. You would start to see and feel results and that would keep you motivated. The better you got at yoga, the more you would probably like it. But all of that would happen only if you didn't give up after the first attempt or two. You can probably think of at least one time in your life when you were ready to give up just before events took a turn for the better, so use that example as an incentive. The following story is a great example of what can happen when you focus on the positive instead of the negative.

Charlotte, one of the women in the Winners' Circle, said she didn't learn to give herself credit for her small victories until her therapist helped her to acknowledge how much blame she took for her "small failures." She said, "I could get a hundred things done in a day, but if I went to bed and remembered one thing that I didn't get done, I felt like the whole day was a waste. I was the same way with compliments and criticism. I could have a day where ten different people told me I looked great, but if one person asked me something like how much more weight I was going to lose, the other ten people's compliments would disappear from my mind and all I could think about for the rest of the day—and sometimes the next day or two—was that this one person thought I still looked fat. Learning to pay as much attention to the good things as I used to pay to the bad has been the hardest part of keeping the weight off. It's funny in a way, because I had always thought of myself as a positive person! If I hadn't learned how to do this before the factory where I worked closed and I lost my job, I think I would have drowned my sorrows in chocolate malts and gained all my weight back and more. Instead, I forced myself to hang on and keep my attention on the things in my life that I was grateful for, and a couple months later I was able to get another job that paid more and had better benefits."

The next time you're in a situation that you feel like you will never make it out of, think to yourself, "Don't quit five minutes before the miracle!" The more experience you get, the better you will become at climbing over or going around the big obstacles. As Amy says, "No matter how hard it is in the beginning, the key to succeeding is to remember that the longer you keep it up, the easier it will get."

An important part of building your emotional muscles is learning to be your own cheerleader. When you first start praising or complimenting yourself, it's normal to disagree with what you just told yourself. It's like a knee-jerk reaction. You don't have to suffer from schizophrenia or have a multiple personality disorder to feel like there are sometimes two different opinions in your head at the same time. For instance, when you're practicing complimenting yourself, you might look in the mirror, smile, and say, "That jacket looks really good on you." Then the other voice pipes up and says, "Your hair looks terrible," or maybe "You're not going to look really good until your stomach is flatter." Don't let that other voice—the inner critic—discourage you. Keep practicing giving yourself praise, because after a while you will begin not only to appreciate it, but will hopefully realize that it's true!

By being your own cheerleader, you will learn that there's a big difference between what you *know* is true and what you *feel* is true. For instance, you know that by doing certain things and not doing others, you'll be able to maintain your weight. But unless you feel the truth of that, you may still feel depressed, discouraged, or fearful of what you're facing. On the flip side of that coin are the people who feel they can keep the excess weight off, even if they go back to their old habits or don't come up with a solid game plan for how they are going to succeed. Both of those examples illustrate what Amy calls "feelings versus facts."

Most people experience this gap between what feels true and what is true from time to time, but people who have made huge changes in their life sometimes have this conflict come up more often because they are still getting used to the changes that they've made.

When you're feeling stressed out or have a lot of anxiety about something, the gap can get even bigger. When that happens, unless you train yourself to find out the facts, you will probably believe that whatever you're feeling or fearing is true. For example, Mariah, a woman in the Winners' Circle for five years, said that when she was losing weight, she used to participate in a weekly conference call with other people who were using the same weight loss program. After she lost forty pounds, the woman who organized the conference calls asked her if she would be willing to talk about her experience. The conference call was usually about forty-five minutes long and Mariah was scheduled to be the last presenter for that week. She said, "I started telling my story and after about five minutes I heard a beep on the line. Then I heard another beep and another and then a bunch of beeps, one right after the other. I thought the beeps meant that people were hanging up and I started to sweat and feel like I must be boring people, so I cut a bunch of details out of the story and wrapped it up. I felt terrible the whole next day. I was so embarrassed about how bad my presentation was that when the lady who organized the call left me a message I was afraid to call her back. When I finally got up the nerve to call her, she said, 'Everyone really liked what you shared last night, including the people who were coming on line for the next call. I wish you wouldn't have cut it short!' I was stunned. I said, 'I thought people didn't like it since I heard all those beeps. I thought people were hanging up.' She said, 'You don't hear a beep when people hang up, only when a new person comes onto the line.' I felt relieved and really silly!"

When you're feeling upset, worried, afraid, or any negative emotion, practice putting aside what you're feeling for a few minutes and ask yourself, "What factual evidence do I have to support this feeling?" (I can now say that I've learned what the word "fear" really stands for: False Evidence Appearing Real.) If you and I have anything in common—and we obviously do—you will probably be shocked by how many times you "feel sure" something is true, even though you have no real evidence to back up that feeling. Stopping yourself and checking to compare feelings with facts is an important exercise for building your emotional muscles.

Another important exercise is to learn to stop yourself when you start beating yourself up and turn your attention to the things you've done well. For instance, even if you've had a day of bingeing, you can prevent the domino effect and limit the damage by stopping to appreciate yourself for doing really well for the past ten days or however long it's been. Being willing and able to feel grateful to yourself for all the work you've done and what you've achieved so far is an important part of sticking with your game plan and keeping up your emotional strength. Amy says, "Giving yourself credit and appreciating yourself for the changes you've made can solidify your sense of self-esteem and give you the power to keep going. The less gratitude you have for yourself and the more you beat yourself up, the less control you'll have the next day, and you don't want to do that to yourself." Focusing on the ten strong days you had in a row, as opposed to the one binge day, will keep you on track. Imagine if you hadn't had those ten days. Count the good days, not the bad! They will add up.

Practicing patience is absolutely vital at this stage. (I'm glad I was never a doctor because I used to have no patience!) Many people in the Winners' Circle say they have gotten good at having patience with other people and that is an accomplishment worth celebrating! But most people would benefit by learning how to be more patient with themselves. For example, Paul, a fifty-two-year-old supervisor at a home for people who are developmentally disabled, has the patience of a saint with the people who live there and the people he works with each day. But he says that treating himself with as much patience as he has for others feels uncomfortable to him. He said, "When I don't get as much done as I think I should have or when it takes me more than a couple minutes to figure something out, I can feel my blood pressure rising, and before I know it I'm swearing at myself and banging things around in the office. And then I get mad at myself for being mad at myself. I never treat anybody else like that, but I can't seem to stop doing it to myself."

HOT TIP

The Fountain of Youth

Tell me I need to drink eight to ten glasses of water a day and I say yuck, I need flavor! I am a big baby!

Tell me all the health benefits you can think of. Tell me I'll have healthier organs or a longer life and it still won't get me to drink more water. On the other hand, find something that really matters to me, and voilà! You will have me drinking water all day long. In my case, finding out that water will make my skin more gorgeous and youthful was enough to start me drinking. With each sip I imagine flawless skin and all the wrinkles being plumped out. Okay, so vanity is my insanity, but it works!

Find something that will make drinking water appealing to you, because you really do need to drink about a quart of it for every fifty pounds of body weight. If plain water doesn't do it for you, make it taste better by adding some apple, lemon, lime, orange, or cucumber slices. Figure out what floats your boat and get in the water game!

Like Paul, I also struggle with learning to have more patience with myself and for situations in general, but I can celebrate how far I've come! Many years ago I was staying in a motel after completing an aftercare program in the South, and in the middle of the night I saw these huge water bugs in the bathroom. I wouldn't touch them and I had to get rid of them so I told my friend, "We have to go to a store and get a broom right now." I wasn't in the store two seconds when I blurted out, "There's no brooms!" I hadn't even looked for them yet. So now I laugh about that and call it the "no-broom mentality." It's what they refer to in twelve-step programs as King Baby. I want what I want when I want it!

Your Accomplishments Are Worth Celebrating

You definitely have accomplishments that are worth celebrating, and if you look at each day closely and with an open mind, you can find personal growth and achievements in every area of your life, not just in your fitness and nutrition!

Whereas your small victories are the meaningful molehills that you overcome every day, your accomplishments are the goals that you are committed to striving for, like exercising a certain number of times each week, being more accountable to the promises that you make to yourself and others, learning to have more patience for yourself, and being willing to stretch your comfort zones to try new things.

Every day is another step away from feeling out of control and toward feeling safer and more confident that you can stay in control, at least most of the time. When you look at each little change you've made separately, it may not look like much, but when you put them all together, you can see that you've taken giant steps toward living a longer, healthier, and happier life. (I like to think of it like stringing a pearl necklace, putting one pearl on the strand for every positive change to make a gorgeous accessory.)

Take a few minutes right now to review the accomplishments that you've already made. Open your Winners' Circle Workbook and list ten things that you've accomplished since you first began to lose weight. You are going to be amazed by how much you've already done that you haven't acknowledged or appreciated. So take a bow and give yourself a standing ovation! Each time you reach another goal, add it to your list and celebrate your accomplishment!

Accomplishments from the Winners' Circle

Since people have a way of downplaying their own accomplishments, these examples from the Winners' Circle should help you to remember and recognize more of the things that you have accomplished or remind you of goals that you want to accomplish.

No More Sneak Eating

Everyone in the Winners' Circle can celebrate the accomplishment of giving up sneak eating. They eat what they crave in public and they are their own judges and juries. Regardless of what many people believe, they have discovered that sometimes having what they crave is the smartest thing they can do. Eating what they crave in public also helps them to refrain from overdoing it. For instance, Patrick, who has been in the Winners' Circle for more than ten years, said, "Every once in a while I just have to have a cheeseburger, and I let myself have one." He says he eats a cheeseburger a couple times a month, on average. He just makes sure that the rest of his nutrition and fitness game plan is on track so his two cheeseburgers satisfy his craving without causing any weight gain.

Rebounding Quickly from a Binge

An accomplishment that is very worthy of celebration is the ability to rebound quickly from a binge. Members of the Winners' Circle know that one binge isn't going to do them in, and they celebrate the accomplishment of learning how to get right back on track immediately after it. Being able to do that gives them much more confidence and serenity. Patty, who has been in the Winners' Circle for more than three years, said, "Learning to nip a binge in the bud has made all the difference for me. It used to be that when I was on a diet, one piece of pie was all it took for me to spin out of control. I'd be back to a pie a day for months before I could get myself to quit again. Now I let myself have a piece of pie every once in a while, but I know that it's just one piece. If I end up eating half the pie, I throw the other half away or give it to someone before I can eat any more and I go out and walk a few miles. I tell myself that the walk is damage control, and when I get back home I acknowledge myself for being back on track."

Setting and Keeping Smart Boundaries

Learning to set reasonable boundaries for yourself and keep those boundaries is an accomplishment that benefits you in all areas of your life and is totally deserving of celebration! (When I was at my heaviest I had no boundaries whatsoever and people called me on it all the time.) Your ultimate goal is to be able to set and keep smart boundaries on your own, but there's nothing wrong with getting other people to help you practice until you get good at it! You can also make a game of it to make it more fun. For example, when I go to a salad bar, I use a small plate instead of a dinner plate, and I allow myself to pile the salad as high as I want. But I don't allow myself to eat anything that falls off the plate or go back for seconds.

Maynard, a member of the Winners' Circle for four years, said that it was easy to set boundaries, but keeping them, especially when he was traveling, was very hard for him to do. He said, "There were months when I was traveling so much for my business that I was away more than I was home and I was taking clients out to dinner three or four times every week. I always knew what I should order, but I couldn't seem to do it. I would have the word 'salad' on the tip of my tongue and then order the French fries instead. When I told my wife what I was doing, she said, 'Why don't you call me when you place your order, and maybe that will give you incentive to order what's good for you?' I didn't want to look ridiculous in front of my clients, so I used to pretend I had a message from her and was just giving her a quick call back to let her know I'd call her after dinner. I would hit the speed dial button and time it so she was on the line when I gave the waiter or waitress my order. It worked like a charm." Jonathan, a member of the Winners' Circle for two years, says that during the first year that he was maintaining his weight loss, he had to avoid parties because he couldn't stop himself from overindulging in just about everything. He said, "The fact that I can go to a party, choose two things that are normally off-limits for me, and enjoy those things without feeling deprived because I'm not stuffing everything on the dessert table into my mouth is a huge accomplishment for me. My strategy is to look at everything that's on the table and then do a little informal research to figure out what is most worth using the calories on. I take my sweet tooth very seriously! I walk around and talk to people and I ask them if what they're eating is really good. Doing the research gives me a chance to talk to people I know and meet people I don't know. It also slows me down and helps me get over the initial head rush of seeing all those tempting desserts in one place. After I decide which two treats I'm going to have, I space them out so I'll have one about an hour after I get to the party and plan to have the other one at least an hour later. If my second choice is gone by the time I go back to the table, sometimes I choose something else, but a lot of times I'm happy to walk away without picking an alternate because I know I'm saving calories and usually by that point in the party I'm having enough fun without the extra fat or sugar that I really don't miss it."

HOT TIP

Time to Glow!

One of the small victories that I enjoy most is the glow I get from taking care of my skin. By investing just a few minutes each morning and every night,

I can delay the effects of aging and put my best face forward.

If you haven't considered how much improving your skin can lift your spirits and boost your self-esteem, you might be surprised at how much joy a simple skin care routine can add to your day. People who have had bad nutrition habits often have skin that doesn't look healthy and vibrant, but now that you are eating healthy foods and exercising, it won't take that much effort to renew your skin's condition and give off a youthful radiance.

The secret to beautiful skin is to find a skin care routine that works for you and stick with it. You will get immediate results, and that will be very gratifying. We are so lucky that we live in an age where there are products that can dramatically improve our skin and significantly delay the signs of aging. Thank God the days of our mother's cold cream are gone. To get the most for your money, don't fall for fancy packaging, shop for the best ingredients. Be sure to always apply moisturizer with SPF 30 before putting on your makeup. To make expensive serums last longer, you can mix them with a bit of over-the-counter moisturizer. Look for products with higher levels of hydroxyl acids and vitamin C. Hydroxyl acids exfoliate dead skin cells and help to fade sun spots, making your skin smoother and younger looking. Vitamin C stimulates the natural development of collagen, reduces lines and wrinkles, helps to prevent future wrinkles due to sun and free radicals, and gives your skin a radiant glow.

I use a glycolic acid moisturizer at night for one full week, and then the next week I use a vitamin C moisturizer instead. Alternating the two ingredients like that has produced results that I feel very good about.

Practicing Moderation

Learning to practice moderation is an achievement that just about everyone in the Winners' Circle is proud of and happy to celebrate. Since we were all overeaters for part or most of our lives, the word "moderation" in relation to food wasn't even in our vocabulary, let alone part of our lifestyle. Personally, I used to be completely puzzled by moderate eating. I couldn't comprehend it. I used to make a joke whenever I'd see somebody come out of Dunkin' Donuts with just one doughnut and cup of coffee. I'd say, "Why did that man get out bed? Why did he turn the key in his car? Why did he even bother to walk through that door?" I couldn't believe that somebody would go into a store to get *one* doughnut. People in the Winners' Circle celebrate finding pleasure in small treats and know that practicing moderation is another form of maturity.

Getting Real and Getting More Real

You have to be real with yourself if you're going to keep winning after losing. For example, if you think you've done well for the past week, but you get on the scale and you've gained three pounds, you have to be willing to take an honest look at what you were doing and not doing for the past seven days. To get a true sense of what's happening if you think you might be getting off track, you may want to keep a food and exercise diary. For a lot of people, keeping a daily food and exercise diary is part of their game plan for life and it works great for them. Other people only keep the diary when they gain a few pounds because keeping it every day makes them focus too much on food. Everyone is different, so it's really important to figure out what works best for you and keep making adjustments that keep you winning. (When I gain, I take an honest look at what I'm eating. Sometimes I had tuna and pickles or other foods with too much salt and I know it's water retention and can quickly make that adjustment.)

The important thing is to get real and continue to get more real with yourself. Burying your head in the sand isn't going to help you maintain your weight unless there's nothing to eat under there! Maintaining isn't about coasting. It's about staying on top of your game and as soon you see that you've put on a few pounds, taking them off again.

George, who has kept twenty-five pounds off for more than five years, said, "In the past when I lost weight, I'd always gain it back because I'd tell myself that I could have a big piece of pie or a huge bowl of ice cream because I exercised that day. I knew that walking a couple of miles didn't burn off enough calories to make up for that much dessert, but I didn't want to accept the truth, so I'd keep selling myself that story until I couldn't buckle my belt. And then I'd have to go back to square one and lose the weight all over again. Finally, I admitted to myself that come hell or high water I was going to eat something really fattening at least once a week. That reality meant that for me to avoid regaining my weight, I'd have to figure out how many more calories I really had to burn off because walking a couple miles a day sure as hell wasn't enough!" Now George runs an average of five miles a day, swims for thirty minutes three times a week, carefully monitors his calorie intake every day, and gets to have his big dessert once a week without gaining weight. There are plenty of rewards and payoffs for being real with yourself!

Another very valuable part of being real with yourself is knowing when it's time to make another change. Let's say you've been running a couple miles a day and doing weight training three times a week, but you notice that your clothes are starting to feel a little tight, and the scale tells you that you've put on a few pounds; or maybe your size and weight are in great shape, but you just feel bored and notice that your motivation is slipping. Those are clear signs that it's time to do something different by either changing your exercise routine or your eating habits, or maybe trying something new to add some spice back into your life.

Growing in Comfort, Confidence, and Self-Respect

It's a victory to change your posture and body language from shutting people out to inviting them in. It's also a victory to discover that when you were overweight, people weren't avoiding you because of your size. People who don't feel comfortable about themselves typically carry themselves a certain way. They tend to walk with their heads down, their eyes downcast, and their bodies closed in, instead of walking tall, smiling, and making eye contact. Everything about the low self-esteem body posture says, "Don't talk to me." Many people who have lost weight say they didn't want to meet new people when they were heavier because they didn't feel like they were presenting who they really were. Nearly all of the people in the Winners' Circle say they feel "more like themselves" at their healthy weight than they ever did when they were heavy. The real self was always in there for all of us; we just had to find a way to bring him or her out.

The better you feel about yourself on the inside, the easier it is to express those good feelings on the outside. Dr. Nadler explains, "The body will exhibit what the mind is thinking and what you are feeling emotionally. In order to continue growing your confidence level and increasing your self-respect, it's important to give at least as much time and attention to your positive character traits and qualities as you give to the things you consider faults. One way to do this is to practice deleting self-critical thoughts and instantly replacing them with thoughts that are more affirming. For example, when you catch yourself thinking something like, 'I look terrible,' practice instantly replacing that thought with something that you believe is sincerely positive about your appearance, such as, 'My hair looks nice,' or 'This top looks good on me.'" The same thing will work with your emotions. She says, "If you're going to a party and catch yourself thinking, 'I'm just not very interesting to talk to,' replace that thought with, 'Everyone has something interesting about them, including me.'"

Dr. Nadler explains, "Typically, if we honestly and objectively examine ourselves, we can find plenty of good qualities, but often we have spent so much time reinforcing what we don't like that at times we have difficulty finding what we do like and sometimes it takes a while to get comfortable expressing those qualities. It's important to have at least one person in your life who can be your 'phone a friend' lifeline. Choose someone who is a reliable source for positive feedback and who you know wants you to win and knows how to help you refocus on your good qualities that make you feel better about yourself. While I recommend that you learn how to become your own champion, if you are having trouble, this member of your support team can be just a phone call away. Your job, once they reveal something wonderful about you, is to accept it and then just 'act as if.' If you want to exhibit more confidence, but aren't feeling confident, try acting as if you are. In time, you will actually start to feel more confident, and the more practice you get, the more natural it will feel, until you are, in fact, confident. The idea is similar to the way we can make ourselves feel happier by smiling. When we first put that smile on our face, we may not feel happy at all, but the physical act of smiling eventually sends the message to our brain that we're feeling good, and then suddenly we realize that we *are* feeling good. And remember, it takes three times as many muscles to frown as it does to smile. So why not save your energy for working your whole body out and give your face a break?"

GOOD-BYE FAT, HELLO FRIENDS!

Before Marissa lost the forty pounds she'd put on after high school, she used to dread running into anyone from her hometown. She said, "When I graduated, I weighed 110 pounds and wore a size 6. While I was away at college I put on about fifteen pounds, and then when I started my new job I gained another twenty-five pounds in just a few years. I'm only five foot three, so forty extra pounds made me look like a beach ball with fat little arms and legs sticking out. I used to go straight home after work, except for pit stops at fast-food drive-thrus. I went grocery shopping in the middle of the night so I wouldn't run into anybody I knew, and I never went out to the mall or anywhere else. If I was walking down the street (which I rarely ever did) and saw people up ahead that I knew, I would practically dive into whatever store I was in front of to avoid having to talk to them and have them see me that way. Now that I've lost weight and feel good about myself I look forward to running into people from high school. It's funny because I did such a good job of hiding that most of the people I run into think I just moved back to this area. They have no idea I've been hiding out here all along!"

The Joy of Simple Pleasures

To win after losing, it's important not only to appreciate and celebrate your accomplishments, but also to learn how to notice and feel grateful for all of the simple pleasures that are part of everyday life. Opening up to joy is a way of feeding your mind and your heart. When you were losing weight, you learned how to slow down and be more aware and present with your food, and now it's time to slow down and be more aware of all the wonderful things that are around you. I never noticed all the things I notice now when I was in my addiction mode. Now I can literally stop and smell the roses, and so can you! Pet a dog, watch children play, go under a sprinkler, enjoy the shade of a tree and the colors of a sunset. Take the time to appreciate the skill and artistry of a painting or piece of jewelry. The idea is to take in all the things that make you happy and let them warm and feed you. That way you won't feel the need for the extra calories to feed you.

Can you imagine what the world would be like if everyone noticed and talked about all the little things they like as much as they notice and talk about all the little things they don't like? It's incredible that people spend so much time complaining when they could be sharing their happiness, appreciation, and excitement, if they only tuned in to the positive things instead of the negative. I've learned to walk away from negative people in a polite way. If they tell me how horrible things are I try to point out something good, then I say, "Have a nice day," and move on. Negative people are like gum. They try and stick to you. I say, spit out the gum and go get a lifesaver! So I am inviting you to start noticing and feasting on the simple joys and pleasures of everyday life, the way you used to notice and feast on your favorite foods. Start a list of "Simple Pleasures" in your Winners' Circle Workbook and challenge yourself to add at least one item to your list every day.

To get you started, here are some of the simple pleasures that people in the Winners' Circle appreciate and celebrate:

Fresh-cut flowers. (I buy them every week!)
The way I look in my clothes.
Sorbet and Italian ice—who knew fat free could be
    so good!
Leaving my fat nicknames behind.
Smiles and compliments from cute guys.
Having a lap for my grandson to sit on.
Being able to climb stairs without losing my breath.
Playing with my grandchildren.
Shopping in the petite department!
Running without my butt bouncing.
Having twentysomething guys stop and talk to me.
Singing in my synagogue's choir and blowing the
    shofar.
Being able to have chocolate in the house without
    eating it.
Feeding the birds.

COUNT EVERY DAY AS A VICTORY!

Up until eight years ago, Ginger could have been the poster girl for yo-yo dieters. Now she has the honor of having been featured in one of Jenny Craig's national commercials. She said she lost and gained weight throughout her life too many times to count but knows that she gained and lost between 700 and 800 pounds during thirty years of yo-yo dieting that began with her first Weight Watchers meeting when she was only ten years old.

She said, "I started the Jenny Craig Weight Loss Program in April of 1997 and weighed 269 pounds at the time. On February 13, 1999, I hit my goal weight of 144 pounds. After a lifetime of struggle, I was a new person and I had gotten my life back. Every day since then, more than 2,920 days, has been a victory. I was thrilled when I won the battle of losing my weight, but I knew that maintaining the weight loss would be my real triumph."

She said, "I don't deny myself food. I found through the years of yo-yo dieting that when I would not let myself eat or not allow myself to have something I really wanted, I couldn't stop thinking about it and then, oh my gosh, look out! I pitied the person who got in my way of the refrigerator. I never will forget how I used to deny myself a slice of cake at a birthday party and then buy an entire birthday cake and binge-eat it when no one was around. After being a yo-yo dieter for so long and living in the dark tunnels of defeat, finally finding my way to the end of the tunnel, where the light beamed on me brightly, was like being born all over again. It has made me appreciate every minute of every day. I don't take anything for granted. My entire outlook has changed. My entire life revolves around one idea that I adapted for myself: 'Live life, love it, and be the best that you can be.'"

THE IMPERFECT TEN

The Top Ten Small Victories Worth Celebrating

1. Being able to see your feet when you're standing up.
2. Ordering a salad or a veggie or turkey burger instead of a beef burger because that's what you really want and you know that eating less fat makes you feel better.
3. Finding lingerie in your favorite color that shows off your "bling" and hides everything else.
4. Becoming an approachable person by changing your body language a little at a time. (Next time you go to your local café or coffee shop, leave the laptop at home. People are more likely to start a conversation if your head is not buried in a project.)
5. Being able to take a compliment without saying something negative back. A simple thank-you will do.

6. Deciding what time you will exercise instead of *if* you will exercise.

7. Feeling good about saying no to certain foods, instead of feeling deprived.

8. Going to the beach or pool because you love it, no matter how your body looks.

9. Achieving greater serenity with food, instead of having to count every single calorie or fat gram that goes into your mouth every single day.

10. Doing things that you love doing for no special reason other than that they make you feel happy.

STEP 5

Stay in the Game
You Have to Play to Win

*I count him braver who overcomes his desires than him
who conquers his enemies; for the hardest victory is the
victory over self.*

—Aristotle, *Stobaeus Floritigium*

No matter how good your maintenance game plan is or
how successfully you're dealing with the emotional challenges in your life, chances are that you will hit some bumps
in the road. Whether those bumps are "bad"—like disappointments or disasters—or "good"—like being promoted
or starting a new relationship—if you don't have some solid
coping skills, they can throw you for a loop and cause you
to make some unhealthy choices. To land on your feet, you
need a plan for when your plan fails.

There have been lots of bumps in my life since I lost
weight, and I hardly ever saw them before I ran into them.
Some of the bumps have been so big they almost knocked

me out. When my boyfriend broke up with me and later declared that his new girlfriend was only 110 pounds soaking wet, I felt like he had punched me in the stomach. When one of my varicose veins burst open and I almost bled to death, the terror that my life would end just as I was starting to enjoy it just about floored me. When my first plastic surgeon, Dr. Mark, who had given me my life back, died of cancer in his early forties, I was so sad that I barely made it through the first couple of months after hearing about it. When things like that happened, I found out that my basic game plan for maintaining my weight just didn't cut it.

So this chapter includes as many things as the experts and I could think of that will help you to stay in the Winners' Circle when you have to deal with situations or circumstances that are too big for your basic game plan to handle. You'll put together your own emergency Bag of Tricks and find out how to beat the Big Ds—decisions, deadlines, disappointments, and disasters. In other words, you're about to learn how to hit a curveball!

If you expect maintenance to be easy sailing, the first big wave that hits you will not only rock your boat, it will probably capsize you. On the other hand, if you know that hard times and challenges are part of life for everyone, you won't take it so personally when things go wrong, and instead of getting stuck in the problem, you can focus on finding a solution. As the old saying goes, "Smooth seas do not make skillful sailors." Typically, it's not the easy days that make you stronger and wiser, it's the difficult days. The biggest breakdowns can lead to the biggest breakthroughs, if you stay in the game.

If you haven't already committed to staying in the game "no matter what," now is the time to make that promise to yourself. It's the one vow you must make and continually renew to stay in the Winners' Circle. Take out your Winners' Circle Workbook and put that promise in writing right now. As you will read in this chapter, it's okay to take a planned and structured "time-out" when you really need one. It's even okay to slip off the wagon once in a while. What is not okay, what is a definite deal-breaker, is to let that slip keep you down. One of the best insights from the Winners' Circle is that when you know and accept that there are going to be times when you want to give in and give up, you have more power and options for dealing with those times.

Winning When You're Down

A curveball catches a batter off guard because he thinks the ball is heading one way and then without warning it changes direction and goes somewhere else. The same thing can happen with events and situations in your life. You think things are going one way, you're ready to deal with them as they appear, and then without warning they change. When the change is for the worse, it can drain a lot of your energy and trigger your old desire to decompress, numb out, and soothe yourself with food. When the change is for the better, it can make you feel elated and pumped up and trigger a desire to celebrate with food.

Learning to hit a curveball is learning how to take care of your physical and emotional needs when you're upset or feeling down without resorting to eating unhealthy foods or overeating. When you hit a low point, Amy says that it's very important to find something that appeals to any of your five senses, except taste. Think about what will make you feel good that involves your sense of touch, smell, sight, or hearing. To stimulate your sense of touch, get a massage or a pedicure, soak in a warm bath, or take your time smoothing lotion or oil all over your body. For your sense of smell, there are all sorts of wonderful sources of aromatherapy, including scented candles, putting on your favorite perfume, trying new perfumes, or buying yourself flowers. To stimulate your sense of sight, go to a museum, art gallery, or even a store and look at the things that you like. For me, a bright-colored feather boa heightens my sense of sight and touch because it just feels so good around my neck. One of the women in the Winners' Circle said she loves to go into quilt shops because it's fun to see all the different fabric patterns and the creative and original way people put them together, even though she doesn't do quilting or even sew. If you can't get out, sometimes just flipping through magazines or catalogs can do the trick.

If you're most into your sense of hearing, listen to your favorite music. Music can rock your world and help you to tune in to feelings that you don't even know you're having. Another way to stimulate your sense of hearing is to tune in to radio stations that you've never listened to before, just to

hear something new or different. Or go to a beach and tune in to the rhythm of the waves and the sounds of the seagulls. If you can't get to the beach, you can get the beach DVD at Bed, Bath and Beyond. It brings the beach to your living room. (Sexy lifeguards not included!)

When you want to satisfy your taste buds without eating, have a tea ceremony for yourself. Brew your tea in a pretty teapot and sip it from one of your favorite cups. It smells good, it tastes good, and the warmth will help you to feel good. Choose a tea that goes with how you're feeling, or select one that will help to support the way you want to feel. If you want to wake up and feel more energized, try a mint tea. If you want to calm down and relax, try something like orange spice, decaffeinated chai, or one of the teas labeled as "calming." It always makes me feel like I'm a little girl having a tea party, and that appeals to me.

If your thoughts keep going back to soothing yourself with sugar or fattening foods, force yourself to wait at least thirty minutes before you give in to the temptation. (Trust me, the cupcake will wait.) One of the best ways to fill those thirty minutes is with exercise or some sort of physical activity. If you exercise, dance, or even vacuum or dust for a half hour, you will feel better about yourself, your body will release more endorphins, and you probably won't be as hungry or have the same urge to pig out afterward. Drinking a large glass of water or two after you exert some physical effort will help you to feel full and increase your energy level. (Unsweetened decaffeinated ice tea works well, too.) Exercise is

one of the things you can count on to automatically change your emotional state. Accept that you probably won't want to do it when you're feeling down and out, and then do it anyway because it's certain to make you feel better.

If after thirty minutes of doing something physical you still honestly feel like you need to indulge in something decadent, first play the substitution game. Decide what you most want to eat and then see if you can re-create it as a less guilty pleasure. If you're craving a chocolate ice cream cone, will a fat-free Fudgsicle do the trick instead? If your mouth is watering for a piece of apple pie, will a sliced apple, drizzled with a little honey, agave nectar, or maple syrup satisfy the urge?

If after all of that you still feel like you're going to have an emotional meltdown unless you go to Dairy Queen or Dunkin' Donuts, then go. But only if you can go without guilt! Amy says that in a real crisis, who cares if you binge? She says, "A one-time binge is not going to ruin your whole game plan. The thing is to let it happen without beating yourself up. If you recognize that every once in a while this is going to happen, you don't fall into the mind-set of thinking that you screwed up and therefore might as well binge for the next three weeks."

She also says that anything you can do to limit the damage is useful, but the key is to not keep repeating this behavior. She says, "If you're going to binge, it's almost always better to go out to eat than to stay home, because when you're in public you're less likely to go crazy. If you can,

invite someone to go with you. That way, you can treat yourself without going to town in the shame zone, which is what happens when you're sitting by yourself eating entire bags of potato chips, half gallons of ice cream, or whole pizzas."

Ready for another life-changing tip from the Winners' Circle? If you binge or splurge, do not skip your exercise that day. Go to the gym or wherever you exercise as soon as you can get there. If you do this, I promise you that you will maintain instead of gaining. And you will win by losing the old mind-set that there's no point in exercising after you've splurged and blown your calorie total for the day. That's actually one of the best times to exercise because it changes your mood, stops the binge from taking you over, and keeps you from doing more damage physically and emotionally. Skipping your workout after a binge is adding insult to injury and pounds to your body. If you want to be absolutely certain that you won't feel guilty after a binge, then decide what you're going to eat, figure out how many calories your binge will cost you, and work them off *before* you indulge!

Is There a Better Choice I Can Make?

Sometimes you will need to have a treat. Most people can't just give something up completely, so you either need to learn how to satisfy your temptations with smaller portions, find healthier substitutes, or do both!

Since those times are sure to come up, it's a good idea to have some smart alternatives that feel decadent and taste delicious, but won't break the calorie bank. After reading the list of my favorite healthy replacements below, make your own list of your biggest temptations. Then go to the library or get online and do the research for replacement items that are healthier choices but still satisfy your taste buds. (E-mail me some; I always like to add to my list!)

Bagel

> **(2.5 oz. = 250+ calories)**
> > **with regular cream cheese (1 Tbsp. = 55 calories)**
> > **(251 or more total calories)**
> Scoop out the bagel (about 50 calories) and adorn it
> with no-fat (1 Tbsp. = 20 calories) or light cream cheese
> (1 Tbsp. = 35 calories) and two tomato slices (about
> 20 calories). (Total calories for substitution = 105 or less.)

Slice of Cake

> **(350 to 500+ calories)**
> Fat-free angel food cake. Add fresh strawberries and
> low-fat or fat-free Cool Whip and it's unreal! (About
> 200 calories or less.)

Piece of Candy

> **(1 oz. = from about 22 to 150+ calories)**
> Reach for sweet fruits instead. (1 cup of cherries =
> 74 calories, 1 cup cantaloupe = 53 calories, 1 orange =
> about 62 calories, 1 cup of grapes = 62 to 106 calories,

1 cup of mango = 107 calories.) Beware of sugar-free candy or any product that says "sugar free." Sugar free does not mean fat free and you can still pack on the calories. Also, some sugar substitutes can have the same effect as a laxative if you eat too much of them. So beware the bowl! (About 53 to 107 calories per cup, plus you get the vitamins and minerals.)

Slice of Cheese

(1 oz. = 85 to 115+ calories)
Low-fat mozzarella string cheese is a decent replacement because you can eat it slowly by pulling away the strings. It can be great for an afternoon pick-me-up when your body is craving protein. Low-fat ricotta is also really good and Alpine Lace offers a variety of great options too. If you're avoiding dairy products but really want cheese, try some of the soy cheese or rice cheese alternatives. (72 calories per ounce.)

Chocolate

(1 oz. = 144 calories or more)
Milk chocolate, dark chocolate, and carob all have about the same amount of calories, but depending on how they are combined with other ingredients like sugar and fats, the calorie count can go way up. The advantage that carob and dark chocolate have over milk chocolate is that they both have some health benefits, but that's

not a good reason to get carried away! Try satisfying your chocolate appetite with an 8 oz. glass of low-fat chocolate soymilk (only 70 calories, and you get about 7 grams of protein, about 4 grams of fiber, and about 290 mg of potassium).

Cookie

(30 to 130+ calories for one cookie)
There are loads of sugar-free and fat-free versions of cookies to choose from. Check out specialty stores and stores like Whole Foods, Vitamin Cottage, Wild Oats, and Trader Joe's. (Be sure to read the nutrition label, though, because sometimes it says low-fat but you're only saving a few calories. The total calories always count, and if you can find a few cookies you like that have low calories and low fat, you're set!) One of my favorites is No Pudge! Fudge Brownie Mix. (You can also order it online at www.nopudge.com.) What I love about these brownies is that they are fat free and include special instructions for how to make just one brownie at a time in the microwave. Do I love Mrs. No Pudge or what! You can't miss the box. It has a pink pig on it. All you do is mix vanilla yogurt with the batter. If you make them for company, no one will be the wiser (www.nopudge.com). One delicious No Pudge! fudge brownie has 110 calories and zero fat grams.

Doughnut

(2 oz. = 220 to 350+ calories)
Sorry. There are no substitutes for doughnuts, so you'll
either have to pay the full calorie price or get over it!

Frappuccino with Whipped Cream

(16 oz. = about 260 to 570 calories)
Order a low-fat version with no whipped cream or ask
for a third or a half of the whipped cream that they
normally put on top. By saying "no whip" and nonfat
milk, you can save 150 calories! If you order a 16 oz.
light frap with no whip, the calories will drop to about
200. For an even lower-calorie choice, try a flavored iced
coffee with nonfat milk and no whipped cream, which
can have as few calories as 130 and as few fat grams as
2, depending on which one you order.

Ice Cream

**(½ cup = 145 calories for vanilla to 180 or more
calories for flavors like chocolate peanut butter)**
You can have the same amount of frozen fat-free vanilla
yogurt or a light fudge bar for about 90 calories, or a
Creamsicle for about 45 calories. Check out the sugar-free
and fat-free varieties of ice cream, popsicles made with
fruit and sweetened with fruit juice, soy ice cream, and
assorted low-fat novelties. There are so many delicious
alternatives, there's no excuse not to make the switch!

Slice of Pie

**(1 oz. apple pie = 67 calories; chocolate cream pie =
86 calories; pecan pie = 113 calories)**
Jell-O sugar-free, fat-free pudding in a pie crust with
low-fat whipped cream is a delicious dessert to serve
when you have company. The cook-and-serve pudding is
better-tasting than the instant and the flavor is so intense
your taste buds will have an orgasm. (About 50 calories.)

Snack Bag of Potato Chips

(1 oz. plain = 152 calories)
An ounce of potato chips labeled "light" is usually about
75 calories, and the baked varieties are even less. But
only buy single-serving sizes. Get real! We all know the
family-size bag is for just that—a family. The large chip
bag is a bottomless pit, so avoid it no matter how much
those shopping clubs will save you for buying bulk!
Even if we spend more on less, isn't a longer life worth
the price?

Soda

**(8 oz. of a soda can range from about 80 to 150 calo-
ries and more)**
Mix 4 oz. 100 percent natural fruit juice with 4 oz.
mineral water and enjoy a sparkling, healthy drink
for about 60 calories for an apple juice drink to about
85 calories for a grape juice drink.

Regular Yogurt

> **(6 oz. vanilla = about 150 calories, and more for fruit and other flavors)**
> Light fruit yogurts are around 70 calories for a 7 oz. serving size, and nonfat varieties are around 60 calories for a 6 oz. serving. Spend some time reading labels and trying some different brands and flavors, so you'll know which choices have the least calories and fat grams and the best taste!

You can see that simply by substituting lower-calorie and lower-fat foods and drinks for higher ones, you can dramatically decrease your calorie count for a day, and when you look at an entire week or month, it's obvious that making smart substitutions is a great and easy way to support your maintenance game plan!

SUBSTITUTIONS KEEP ME IN THE GAME!

Jody shed her excess pounds eight years ago and has kept it off ever since. At five foot four, she now weighs 130 pounds and feels comfortable at that weight. She said she weighs herself every Monday morning and whenever the scale reads over 135, she increases her exercise by fifteen minutes a day and decreases her daily calories by 500 until she's back down to 130. She said, "When I first lost weight, my excitement and all the positive feedback I got from other people kept me going. But after about six months, I couldn't pass a bakery without my mouth watering and I would literally spend the rest of the day fantasizing about cake and cookies. It became an obsession. If it wasn't for lower-fat and sugar-free replacements, I'm not sure if I'd still be in the Winners' Circle. Substitutions like Newman's Own low-fat cookies and fat-free Fig Newtons keep me in the game! I don't eat things like that every day, but once a week or so, or whenever I feel like I really need a treat, those are the things I turn to."

Time for Your Own Bag of Tricks

The reality is that the road of life is not always smooth. Most roads have at least a few bumps. Some of the bumps are small and close together, like speed bumps, and some of them are few and far between but they're big enough to really shake you up, especially if you hit one without seeing it first. That's why staying in the game includes anticipating bumps and coming up with a plan for making it over them ahead of time.

Everyone eventually hits bumps. For some people, it's a bunch of small bumps that wear down their dedication. For other people, it's a traumatic life event like a relationship breakup, losing a job, or being transferred to a new location.

For other people, it's a "good bump" that knocks them off their game, like starting a new job or relationship, getting married, or buying or building a new home. For example, when Stephanie, a member of the Winners' Circle for going on five years, got married, she said, "That threw me for a loop with my exercise and food. For a while, I found my weight creeping up again because I was cooking just about every day, making heavy meat-and-potato meals, and doing a lot of relaxing." Stephanie said that once she realized she was putting weight back on, she knew she had to do something about it before it became too overwhelming. She said, "For one thing, I changed the way I was cooking. My husband and I are eating a lot more salads and fruit now than meat, potatoes, and desserts! I also invited my husband to play a game with me called the Fitness Challenge that my daughter Vicki created to help people lose weight and keep it off. Playing the game kept us moving and motivated and now exercise is part of our everyday life. Even when we're traveling, we find a way to exercise. Sometimes that means walking loops around a rest area for thirty minutes or more, but we're both willing to do what it takes to stay healthy and fit."

I hit one of my most challenging bumps about four years after I lost weight. My right knee became stiff, swollen, and very painful. I could hardly stand up without being in extreme pain, and walking was agony. Just when I thought I had things under control, life got very tricky.

Walking two to four miles a day was a vital part of maintaining my weight. When I wanted a special treat like a piece

HOT TIP
Pay More for Less

I love pretzels and I love a bargain. I could buy a jumbo bag of pretzels on sale for 99 cents. The trouble is that if I buy that bag, I'll eat them or torture myself with wanting to eat them as long as they're in my apartment. So I don't buy them. Instead, I reward myself at the end of the day by giving myself permission to buy a snack-size bag of pretzels from the vending machine for 50 cents. At least twenty snack bags would fit into the jumbo bag. You do the math. But it's not that cut-and-dried. If I look at the difference between how many pretzels I'd eat if I had the big bag and how much that overeating would cost me in calories and self-esteem, buying one snack bag at a time is the best choice.

of cake, I would increase my exercise by walking more that day. I was developing a normal, thin person's mind-set! Not being able to walk and finding out that I was going to need knee replacement surgery almost put me into a tailspin. Without being able to walk at least ten thousand steps a day I thought for sure I would gain all my weight back. I started to feel sorry for myself. Why this, after everything else I'd already gone through and had to endure? I also felt sorry for myself because I needed to buy a cane or I wouldn't have been able to walk at all. The cane was a real button pusher. It reminded me of when I weighed the most and was immobile.

Fortunately, not long after I bought the cane, I spent a couple days with one of my friends who always sees the glass as half full. I told her how badly I felt about using my cane and she said, "Stacey, the cane is only temporary. It's like a cast. In fact, why don't you let people sign it?" That was my light bulb moment. My fear of failing turned into new determination to find a way to keep winning. "If it's only temporary," I thought, "then I can deal with it!"

Once I was able to believe that I could get through the knee crisis, I started to think positively again. That's when I decided I needed to go into my old bag of tricks, pull out what used to work for me, and make some adjustments so it would work for me again. The first thing I pulled out of my bag of tricks was my old pedometer. It was time to start counting steps again, instead of miles. The first day I walked nine hundred steps with my cane, and the third day I was up to fifteen hundred. I pulled out some food tricks too and then I was able to start preparing myself for my upcoming knee replacement and make a new game plan.

Put Together Your Bag of Tricks

Being prepared is the key to your ongoing success. In addition to pulling winning thoughts and behaviors out of your old bag of tricks, you can also make a tangible bag of tricks that will be your mental, emotional, and physical first aid kit.

When you're putting together your Bag of Tricks, keep in mind what worked for you when you were losing weight and were highly motivated and think about the new things you can put in your bag to support your goals and help you over the bumps in the road ahead. It really works. You may even surprise yourself and pull out a rabbit!

Think in terms of mind, body, and spirit. You can use a large bag, a box, a basket, or a combination of all of those things. Gather the things ahead of time that can help you get over the bumps when you hit them. To give you some ideas and get you started, I've shared what's in my own bag of tricks. Whenever you use something from your Bag of Tricks, make sure you replace it within forty-eight hours so it will be there when you need it the next time.

Stacey's Bag of Tricks

▌ A list of all the games I play with myself to eat less and burn more calories.

▌ A list of activities that are simple and relaxing and don't take any thought or planning. (When I hit an unexpected low point, nothing comes to mind, so my list is a real lifesaver! This includes sitting on my roof, walking under a sprinkler on a hot day, reading in the park, and taking a bath with all the girly trimmings like scented candles and bubble bath.)

▮ Magazine articles. (I'm always seeing articles in magazines that I want to read but don't have time to read, so I put them in my bag. Reading is very relaxing and can take my mind off of my food cravings.)

▮ A letter from an *Oprah* fan telling me how I've inspired her. (You can include a letter from a friend, secret admirer, or any note that makes you feel good every time you read it.)

▮ My favorite perfume.

▮ A gift certificate for a dinner for two at my favorite healthy restaurant.

▮ The phone numbers of my best friends.

▮ Breath fresheners. (Mouthwash, chewing gum, and mints make my mouth feel fresh and reduce my urge to eat sweets.)

▮ A vibrator.

▮ A massage gift certificate. (Getting a massage can rock my world and certainly make me forget fudge!)

▮ My iPod programmed with inspirational tunes. (When I'm walking in Manhattan and sniffing hot pretzels and sugar-coated nuts on every street corner, the songs on my iPod give me the strength to resist temptation and keep walking. One of my favorite songs is "I Knew You Were Waiting (for Me)," sung by George Michael and Aretha Franklin.)

▮ A slip of paper that says, "Go to Starbucks *now!*"

▮ Low-calorie snacks. (I keep a Zone bar in my bag of tricks and a list of the places near my apartment where I can buy low-fat treats. I love a place called Tasti D-Lite where they have soft-serve ice cream with almost no fat.)

▌ Favorite photos.

▌ Dog biscuits for my best friend. (Making Gertie happy always makes me happy.)

▌ A roll of quarters. (I can hop on a bus and go anywhere in New York City.)

Make sure you have items in your Bag of Tricks that are inexpensive or free! Chances are, you already have many items for your Bag of Tricks in your home right now. If you want to include some things like massages or manicures that aren't cheap, start saving up for them now so you'll be able to afford them by the time you need them. If you have a birthday coming up, consider asking your family and friends to select items from your Bag of Tricks wish list to give you as presents.

DON'T BE A BEFORE OR AFTER, BE A DURING

I like to say I'm a "during" because I consider myself a work in progress. I'm always learning something new and working on making one improvement or another. I don't like to think of myself as an "after" because that makes it sound like I'm done or, worse yet, like I'm a has-been! Nobody wants to be a has-been!

Still, when I'm feeling down, looking at my before photos and comparing them with my "now" photos can give me a really great boost. Some people who have lost weight want to get rid of all the remnants of their past, but I think holding on to a few photos is a great way to remind yourself of how much progress you've made.

Trying on clothes in your new size is another fun thing to do to give yourself a little mood lift when you need one. If you don't want to spend any money, go to a store that carries clothing you don't like or visit a thrift store and only try on things in your size that you know you won't buy. There's nothing like seeing the physical proof of your accomplishment to help you believe that you've come a long way and silence the negative self-talk. Sometimes if silence is golden we want to be rich!

Rebounding from Rejection

Members of the Winners' Circle, both women and men, married and single, agree that sexual roadblocks and dating dead ends really put their maintenance muscles to the test.

Nobody likes rejection, but thanks to Dr. Greer, we can gain some insights into this painful part of life and learn how to look at the situations in a different way so we don't take them so personally. When it comes to being sexually rejected or being rejected after we have a sexual encounter, the first thing Dr. Greer says is, "It's natural for us to take it personally because we were opening ourselves up and being vulnerable—emotionally, physically, or both—and that makes the feelings that go with rejection cut like a knife."

Since sexual rejection is different for single people than it is for people in committed relationships, Dr. Greer is giving us insights and guidance for both.

Let's start with those of us who are dating. Dr. Greer says, "There are a lot of guys who are all about the sexual conquest, so no matter how good the sex is, they still have a tendency to hit and run. Once they score, they're on to the next conquest, and that's not about you at all. It's all about them taking care of their own needs, both ego and sexual. You don't enter the picture. Nowadays, the option for casual sex is also available to women, and although a lot of women might prefer to be in a relationship, there are some women who want to meet their sexual needs without getting into what they feel could be too heavy of an emotional entanglement."

If you were under the impression that someone you were intimate with was interested in developing a relationship with you, the disappearing act can be a rude awakening. That's another reason why it's important to know what you want and what you expect before hopping into bed with someone. If you are really okay with it being "just sex" with no strings attached, then you can enjoy the ride without worrying about what happens or doesn't happen next. But if you're hoping that having sex will seal the deal for a relationship, it's time for a reality check!

Dr. Greer points out, "If you're dating someone for a while and they are giving you real reasons to believe they want a relationship, and then they disappear after having sex with you, you might need to examine the situation a little more closely. Often, it's not your body or your sexual performance that turned someone off, even though you may think that's what it was. It may have been your insecurity or exposing your fears and vulnerabilities at this early stage that caused someone to back off. If you were uncomfortable in the encounter or you expressed concerns over your body or your performance, or you suggested that there are things about you that he or she might not like, most people either don't know how to respond to that or don't want to. And sometimes you tip them off and call their attention to something that they never would have even noticed. It's like a dripping faucet. If you don't know it's happening, it doesn't bother you, but once you know it's dripping, it really becomes annoying. So protect yourself. Make conscious choices about what you talk about and what you share."

She says, "Especially at the beginning of a relationship, many men are concerned about how much effort a potential relationship is going to take. Independent women tend to be concerned about how much of their freedom a man is looking to take away. If you come off like you are going to need constant reassurance or like you have a lot of expectations, people are more likely to back away than to stay. If, now that you've lost weight, you're trying to make up for lost time, you may require much more attention, romance, emotional support, and reassurance than the average guy or gal feels willing or able to deliver."

For those of you who are feeling sexually rejected in a committed relationship, some of the reasons I just mentioned may apply, but according to Dr. Greer there are other things to look at as well. She says, "If you've gotten into a sexual standoff, your partner, unbeknownst to you, may have become anxious, insecure, and inhibited about having sex. If that's the case, it may take a little time to get reacquainted and feel comfortable with each other again. Take the initiative to plan some fun couple time together, and once you've reestablished your intimacy connection, taking the next step into bed should feel much more natural to both of you."

Dr. Greer explains that if you've initiated sex and your partner has turned you down more than a few times, it's possible that your new and improved look has your partner feeling insecure or uncomfortable about his or her own body. If you're in shape now and your partner is not, you may need to provide reassurance that you still find him or her attractive. Or if your partner had been trying to make love when you were heavier and you kept turning it down, maybe he or she is still hurt or holding a grudge. It may be necessary for you to apologize for rejecting their advances and turning your back on their needs in the past. Once you determine what the roadblock is, don't waste any time tearing it down! Sexual intimacy is an important part of keeping a relationship strong and secure, so do whatever it takes, including seeing a therapist together, to reestablish your sexual link."

Beating the Big Ds

Most of the people in the Winners' Circle agree that there are four big things that can knock them off their game plan. They're talking about the big stuff, what I call the Big Ds:

- *Decisions,* like whether to apply for or accept a new job, whether to move, whether to commit to a relationship or decide to end it.
- *Deadlines* that change your regular routine, require a lot of time and energy to meet, and qualify as "make or break" situations that can either have a positive impact or a very negative result if the deadline is missed.
- *Disappointments* that knock the wind out of your sails, like not getting the job or the promotion you deserve and have been counting on, finding out the woman or man you've had your heart set on just isn't into you, not getting approval on a loan to buy a house, and other events of that magnitude.
- *Disasters* include all of the most devastating things you can encounter in life, including, but not limited to, divorce, disease, financial devastation, and death of a loved one.

When you are experiencing one of the Big Ds, one way to reduce your level of suffering is being willing to acknowledge your pain in whatever way you can. People usually think that feeling sorry for themselves is a very negative thing, but Amy explains that "recognizing something painful has happened and that you are experiencing the emotions associated with it is an important part of staying in touch with yourself and being able to move on." Don't try and push the pain away, because if you do, it's going to wait around in the wings and keep getting stronger, until it ends up spoon-feeding you!

If you don't give yourself permission to feel the pain, or if you want someone else to "get" what you're going through and no one seems to understand, that can multiply your suffering and make you that much more tempted to numb out by overeating. If you don't have someone in your life who understands what you're experiencing, then it's even more important to learn how to validate your feelings for yourself. (It is my guess that there will be at least one person who is willing to listen. Thank God for my male gay friends!)

Amy says, "When you're going through hell, the best thing you can do is keep going." She saw that saying on a greeting card years ago and keeps it up on her bulletin board as a reminder. The more times you can say to yourself, "This sucks, but I'm going to get through it," the stronger you will become. What you don't want to think or say to yourself is that you're having this pain because you didn't lose enough weight, or because you've put some back on, or that you're not a good enough person to deserve a pain-free life. No one gets a pain-free life, no matter how many good qualities he or she has.

There's nothing like experience to help you to learn that you can find your way out of hell. If you give up every time

WHEN THE RUG GETS PULLED OUT FROM UNDER YOUR FEET, HOLD ON

Everyone has different reactions when something throws them for a loop. What one person can handle with no problem might be the same thing that sends someone else straight to the pantry. The hardest curveball for me is rejection. Even after all I've gone through and learned, being rejected still rocks my world and shakes up my confidence. When that happens, I have to remember to practice what I preach and hold on. Holding on is an important part of most people's maintenance plans!

One of the biggest disappointments I've had to face was finding out that my first boyfriend since losing weight was bailing out on his promise to accompany me to a big family wedding. When I first mentioned the wedding, he said we'd get a room at the hotel where the reception was being held and we talked about what a blast we were going to have. I was so excited that I was going with a real date and that I was finally going to get to have my first slow dance. I had been dreaming about that moment for years. But when it was time to send in the RSVP card, my boyfriend told me he couldn't go. He said he'd feel too uncomfortable at a social event with so many people he didn't know. I was completely crushed. Devastated, really. I understood that he was dealing with his own issues, but it still felt like rejection to me.

And then something amazing happened. Noah, one of my best friends and the first man I was ever in love with (in my teen years), offered to take me to the wedding. Even though he wasn't my boyfriend and not a real date in the true sense of the word, going with him to the wedding was the best thing that could have happened. He'd known my family for years, felt completely comfortable, and we had a fantastic time. And when the band began to play the first slow song of the evening, Noah took my hand and without saying a word escorted me onto the dance floor. Somehow it seemed like an act of fate that I would end up having my first slow dance with my first love and now one of my best friends. He made it the magical moment that I had always dreamed of.

The moral of the story is that whatever disappointments you end up facing in your life, particularly the ones that feel like they could drive you over the edge, hold on for dear life like you would hold on to a life jacket if you were on the *Titanic*. And just by holding on, something will change and life will suddenly be good again.

you face a challenge or a problem, then you never get to learn that you can survive just about anything, without resorting to your old ways. Each time I get through something painful, my foundation gets stronger. To keep moving through hell, it's best to do as much of your daily routine as you can.

Decide on the minimum that you must do each day and do it. At the very least, pick one productive thing and do that. Even if it's a really small thing, doing it will help you to feel better and give you more energy to do something else. Just keep putting one foot in front of another.

When you find that you honestly can't stick with your daily routine and you're not even doing the minimum, consider taking the Three-Day Time-Out below that Amy helped me to design. She says, "Don't let it go any further than three days because eating right, exercising, and feeling good about yourself will help you to get through a challenging time much better than not doing those things!" As the saying goes, when you get thrown off a horse, the faster you get back on, the better off you will be. So the goal is to get back into your game plan as soon as you can. The very next day is the best possible scenario, but it's unrealistic to expect to win every single match of this maintenance game. Instead, focus on staying in the game and winning more matches than you lose! You just have to believe that if you keep going, you'll keep winning.

The Three-Day Time-Out

Rules:
1. No guilt or beating yourself up.
2. No actions or behaviors that are potentially life-threatening to yourself or others.
3. Write down a clear intention for the purpose the time-out will serve for you.

For example:

I am taking three days to rest and emotionally regroup. I will follow the prescribed plan for the time-out and make choices that will support my commitment to be ready and able to resume my maintenance game plan four days from now.

Day One

Morning (8 a.m.—or earlier—until noon)

- Eat breakfast. If you can't get yourself to eat what you would normally eat for a healthy breakfast, eat a piece of fruit and a few nuts, or a slice of toast with peanut butter and half of a sliced banana, or a cup of yogurt with a handful of almonds. You can also eat a Zone bar or other nutritional meal bar.
- Devote 30–45 minutes (or more if you like) to doing something that you find very soothing and relaxing. This could be taking a leisurely walk, meditating, sitting by a pond or a waterfall, or sitting in the park. It could also be reading, listening to music, creating artwork, or taking a bath.

Afternoon (noon to 6 p.m.)

- Eat a healthy lunch.
- Spend 30 minutes doing something physical to help your body/mind release tension. This could be dancing; playing tennis, basketball, or some other sport;

swimming; walking vigorously; working in your garden; mowing the lawn; horseback riding; or any activity that gets your body moving and occupies your mind. Choose something that you don't typically do as part of your exercise routine.

Evening (6 p.m. to midnight)

▌ Eat whatever you would most love to have for dinner, guilt free.

▌ Allow yourself to have any dessert or treat of your choice.

Day Two

Morning (8 a.m.—or earlier—until noon)

▌ Eat a healthy breakfast, whether you want to or not.

▌ Get 30 minutes of exercise: 10 minutes cardio, 10 minutes flexibility, 10 minutes strength training or a good long walk or swim.

▌ Spend one hour accomplishing something productive. (Thoroughly clean one room of your house, organize your junk drawer, do your laundry, bathe and groom your dog, fill up one shopping bag with items you are willing to donate to charity, or anything productive that will improve your life or someone else's life, or your surroundings. Throwing things away and giving them away is like an internal and spiritual cleansing. I am actually getting to where I love the smell of cleaning supplies, especially lemon Pine-Sol!)

Afternoon (noon to 6 p.m.)

▮ Eat a healthy lunch.

▮ Devote 30–45 minutes (or more if you like) to doing something that you find very soothing and relaxing.

▮ Enjoy up to two cups of any snack you want—guilt free.

Evening (6 p.m. to midnight)

▮ Eat a healthy dinner, whether you want to or not.

▮ Treat yourself to something physically and emotionally soothing. Take a bubble bath, drink a cup of your favorite decaffeinated tea, get a massage, or have an orgasm. If you want or need to be distracted or entertained, watch a favorite comedy or inspirational show or movie, read a chapter in an uplifting or entertaining book, or flip through a favorite magazine. (I always have a supply of *Vogue*!)

▮ Go to bed no later than midnight. One of the biggest secrets to maintenance success is going to bed earlier. Overeaters often stay up late and the later you are up the more you are likely to eat. If you're unable to fall asleep, read or daydream for another 30 to 40 minutes.

Day Three

Morning (8 a.m.—or earlier—until noon)

▮ Eat a healthy breakfast, whether you want to or not.

▮ Get 30 minutes of exercise: 10 minutes cardio, 10 minutes flexibility, 10 minutes strength training.

▌ Spend two hours accomplishing something. (See Day Two for suggestions.)

Afternoon (noon to 6 p.m.)

▌ Eat a healthy, light lunch.
▌ Plan three "safe days" in a row for the next few days. (Safe days are days that are preplanned to guarantee that you stick with your game plan. A safe day can include a visit to a health spa or gym, spending time with a healthy friend who will eat nutritious low-fat meals with you and exercise with you, attending classes for exercise, meditation, yoga, dance, art, music, acting, or whatever you love to do. The objective is to plan your day, from the time you get up till the time you go to bed, to include people and activities that support your decision to feel good, make healthy choices, and enjoy life.)

Evening (6 p.m. to midnight)

▌ Eat a healthy dinner.
▌ Spend one hour doing something for someone else who needs help. This could be volunteering, talking to a friend or two who need encouragement, or walking someone's dog.
▌ Call a supportive friend and share your plans for the safe day you have planned for tomorrow. Ask him or her to check in on you to help you to stick with your plan.

▌ Take 30 minutes to do something that is calming and soothing to your mind and your body. Choose something that allows you to pamper and nurture yourself, such as the Water Healing Transformation Process (see instructions in box below).

▌ Lights out at midnight. (If you are not sleepy by 11 p.m., have a cup of a relaxing nighttime tea like chamomile, valerian root, or Celestial Seasonings Sleepytime tea. If you often have trouble sleeping, buy or make a small pillow [about the size of a book] filled with lavender, or buy an all-natural lavender spray to add the aroma to your sheets and pillow before you go to bed. The scent of lavender is calming and helps many people to sleep. I just sniff the stuff and I feel better.)

THE WATER HEALING TRANSFORMATION PROCESS
By Dr. Denise Nadler

Imagine you are going on a retreat, a little trip away from the tension, stress, and responsibilities of your daily life. Allow for the possibility that you can leave behind your negative thoughts and judgments and allow yourself the opportunity to enter a new place, with a new feeling about who you are and how you typically feel about your body. Now is the time for you to experience your body in a loving, grateful way—exactly as it is at this moment. The process you are about to experience can have a profound effect on how you feel physically, mentally, and emotionally about yourself and about your life.

Make sure you will not be interrupted for at least 30 minutes. This time is just for you. You may choose to take a bath or a shower. If you choose a bath, fill the tub with warm water and add some bubble bath, bath oil, or Epsom salts. You are going to wash away the old negative thoughts and feelings that are not supporting your mental and physical health and replace them with loving thoughts and feelings. Water has been used as a symbol for many things and most commonly in a ritual of a baptism, which is a rebirth of sorts. Allow yourself to give birth to a refreshed and joy-filled you.

Before you begin, take a few minutes to contemplate how amazing your body is! Your brain consists of about 7 million cells. Your heart beats about 72 times per minute, 103,680 times every day, pumping your blood through nearly 100,000 miles of blood vessels to supply oxygen and nourishment to every cell in your body—some 3 trillion of them. In one square inch of your skin, you have four yards of nerve fibers, 1,300 nerve cells, 100 sweat glands, 3 million cells, and three yards of blood vessels. As old cells die, they are replaced by new ones, every second of every minute of every hour of your life. Your body is a miracle and so are you!

Create a peaceful environment. Dim or turn off the lights and light some candles and possibly some incense. Put on music that soothes your soul. Choose a washcloth or sponge and soap that are special, just for this process. Begin by washing your hands and then your face. Be generous with the soap you put on the cloth and gently and slowly wash your body as if you are washing the body of a dear loved one, perhaps your baby or child, or a lovely person for whom you care deeply.

As you are moving the cloth along your skin, imagine that a healing light is radiating from the cloth. Visualize that light sinking into your skin and filling the body part you are washing with healing light and energy. Allow yourself to luxuriate in the sensation of the soft washcloth, the scent of the soap, and the warmth of the water. Breathe deeply, and with each exhale feel your body relaxing more deeply.

To help your mind to stay focused in the present moment and shift your mind-body state, softly repeat statements such as, "I am letting go of my negative thoughts and feelings," "I am embracing myself and my body in a loving way," and "I am worthy of love." Feel free to make up your own affirmations and positive statements and repeat them like you would a prayer or a mantra. If your mind shifts away, tenderly guide it back in to focusing on this practice. For many people, whispering the statements, rather than just thinking them, helps to keep their mind from wandering.

You can use this practice as often as you like. When you are feeling particularly challenged in your life, you may want to do it every day or at least once a week. Keep in mind that you have the power inside you to help transform and heal your body, your mind, and your spirit.

Note from Stacey: If nothing else, at least take a bubble bath and pretend you're Liz Taylor—complete with your hair wrapped up in a towel!

If you are not able to get back on track after a Three-Day Time-Out, don't kid yourself by saying things will get better on their own. Hitting that low point is a clear sign that you have to take better care of yourself and figure out what it is you need right then. If you can't figure that out, or you know what you need to do but can't get yourself to do it, force yourself to get help from a member of your Winning Team or from a coach or a therapist. Just phone someone and make yourself say the words, "I need your help." People who care about you want to help you just as much as you want to help the people you care about. So don't cheat them out of the chance to do something good for you when you really need it.

THE IMPERFECT TEN

The Top Ten Tips to Stay in the Game

1. Reach out to another human when you need help.
2. Be as kind and understanding to yourself as you would be to your best friend.
3. Truly understand that this time you really do not have to go back!
4. Train yourself to get back on track after a binge. (The quicker you can do it, the longer you'll be in the game. And remember, your goal is to be in the game forever!)
5. Make exercise a friend. Stop saying bad things about it as if it's the enemy! You'll start to believe it's a friend when you see and feel how much better it makes you.
6. Be patient with yourself. If you aren't on your way to learning how to do this, get someone to help you.
7. Don't project too far ahead or too far back. The winners stay closest to the here and now.
8. Believe that you are a winner!
9. Stop thinking about your past failures.
10. Put yourself and your health first. You cannot be there for anyone if you are not well, so making yourself number one is the best way to help your loved ones.

STEP 6

Win One Day at a Time

Start Fresh, Finish Strong

*True courage is to do without witnesses
everything that one is capable of
doing before all the world.*

—François Duc de la Rochefoucauld

Winning after losing is about being the best that you can be right now. The secret to success with less stress is planning ahead, but living just one day at a time. It sounds like a contradiction, but it's not. Having a solid but flexible plan for your day gives you peace of mind so you can focus on each thing that you're doing during the day, instead of worrying about whether you'll have enough time to get everything done, or being distracted because you're not sure what you should be doing next. Learning to do this without being too rigid will be a challenge at first.

By wiping your slate clean at the end of each day and making your plans for tomorrow, you finish the day strong and give yourself the best advantage to make tomorrow another win. Going to bed with a clear conscience and a good plan for the next day also helps you to get your beauty sleep. (Boy, do I need that!) When you wake up feeling and looking like you've had a good night's rest, you have the energy and the confidence to start your day fresh!

One of the most demanding schedules I've ever had was when I was in the movie *The Dress Code*. At that time, I weighed more than 500 pounds, and just getting through the day took every bit of energy I had. My days were planned for me, depending on what scenes we were shooting, but I quickly figured out that the unexpected was part of most days, including the endless script revisions that I got each night and had to memorize for the next day. I had to learn how to keep my mind completely focused on what I was doing so I could do the best job possible and make the best use of my time. When I was on camera, my only concern was the scene we were doing. When I was off camera, I was either resting or preparing for my next scene. By doing the movie, I learned that I could do that with real life too. Living in the moment is like being on camera. When I'm living, I'm focused on that moment in time and whatever I'm doing. When I'm planning and preparing for the next day, then all my attention is on that. The movie taught me that no matter how well prepared you think you are, you must always have a plan B.

Step 6 gives you the insights and skills that will help you to live one day at time, instead of getting ahead of yourself or feeling like you're behind. You will learn how to start each day fresh and finish it with satisfaction. You will increase your awareness of the beauty that is hidden in your flaws and begin to appreciate it. You'll discover how to stay open to promising possibilities and how to add more playfulness into your sex life. You will also have a chance to define and refine a new sense of style that fits your new way of living.

Start Fresh, Finish Strong

Treat each day as a new beginning—an empty stage, blank page, clean slate, or whatever analogy works for you. Planning each day with this intention in mind will help you to keep your focus in the here and now. When you're living completely in the present, you don't have fear, guilt, and regret because fear is attached to the future and guilt and regret are linked with the past. And whether you like it or not, all you ever have is this moment. Right now. The people I consider to be winners in life are the people who come closest to living in the moment!

If you plan your day well, making sure you've built in some extra time for the things that you can't predict, you can focus on what you're doing during the day, knowing that if something unexpected happens, you'll be flexible enough to respond in the way that's best for you. Planning time into your day for situations and events that you can't predict gives you the freedom to take advantage of new opportunities and gives you the option to take a breather if you find that you need one.

LIVE IN DAY-TIGHT COMPARTMENTS

Karl, a recovering alcoholic who has maintained his goal weight for more than five years and refrained from drinking alcohol for more than seven years, said, "When I was in recovery one of my counselors told me to live in day-tight compartments. He helped me to see that if I looked too far ahead, what I was facing would seem overwhelming, and if I dwelled on the past, what I lost and all the mistakes I made would drag me down like cement shoes in a swimming pool. I practiced thinking and talking by starting sentences with the word 'today.' I would think, 'Today I can drink water, juice, or soda.' Or I would say, 'Today I can eat three healthy meals and run four miles.' It took practice, but after a few months it became a habit, and I still swear by it."

When you wake up each day, practice thinking or even saying out loud, "Today is a new day." That statement will remind you that you are starting the day fresh, and with the goal of winning one day at a time. You can't always choose what will happen during the day, but you can decide how you will react and respond to the people and events that you encounter. No matter what you did or didn't do yesterday, you can do something different today. The past can influence the future, but it can't predict it or control it. The quality of your day depends on your thoughts and feelings, the choices that you make, and the action steps that you take. I always got a kick out of the saying, "The road to hell is paved with good intentions," because it's so true. We can have all the good intentions in the world, but if we don't actually do something about them, then intentions are all they are. Everyone who has struggled with the question of when to start a diet knows how easy it is to "intend" to do it, prepare to do it, and not do it. In the past, I gained many pounds preparing for the start of a new diet that never came.

If there's something you've been telling yourself you're going to do for days, weeks, or even months, but you're not doing it, it probably means one of two things. Either you think you *should* do it, but don't really want to do it, or you *do* want to do it, but you're afraid to begin or don't know how. Decide which one it is and stop letting your inaction weigh you down. If you believe you should do it because you know it will be good for you or can improve the quality of your life, then find a way to make yourself do it, whether that means asking a friend to gently remind you what you planned on doing, or creating a way to nudge yourself into action. If fear is holding you back, then work with a counselor, therapist, or coach to face and overcome the fear. If it's lack of knowledge that's stopping you, find someone or some resource that can teach you what you need to learn. I once heard someone say that at the end of our lives, it's not the things we did or the mistakes we made that we regret most, it's all the things we *didn't* do. Even if you live past a hundred, life is short, so get on with it!

Finishing a day strong means finishing the day with a sense of sincere satisfaction and some level of serenity. It's every bit as important as starting the day fresh, because if you don't appreciate the beauty of the day, acknowledge the lessons you've learned, and feel good about what you've done, you're probably going to carry some negative feelings into tomorrow. Doing that will sabotage your attempt for a fresh start and set up a vicious cycle that no one can win. I'm not saying that you should put on rose-colored glasses at the end of the day to make yourself feel good. I'm recommending that you get out your Winners' Circle Workbook and spend five minutes listing the things you can be grateful to yourself and others for from the time you woke up until the end of the day.

I should warn you that when people start doing this exercise, a lot of them come down with a serious case of "Ya, buts." They write down something they feel good about, and then their inner critic pipes up with a "Ya, but you didn't do this," or "Ya, but you could have done that better." Trying to ignore the "Ya, buts" is like trying to ignore an eyelash stuck in your eye. (You can "Ya, but" yourself to death, but then you will have a Ya *butt*.) So, if you have a case of "Ya, buts," write those down in your workbook too. Then do your best to look at each one as objectively as you can and decide if it's something that you honestly want to improve

CHANGING YOUR MIND CHANGES
YOUR ACTIONS

If you tell yourself something over and over again, you'll start to believe it. That's why it's so important to change your negative thoughts and self-talk to positive ones. Deanna, a member of the Winners' Circle for three years, says she used to tease one of her friends who believed in doing affirmations. She said, "My friend Carla has these positive affirmation cards all over her house and even in her car. I used to read them out loud in weird and funny voices and we would both laugh. She knew I loved her and wasn't putting her down; I just didn't get the whole New Age thing. She never tried to talk me into doing them and she didn't defend doing them either. One day we were having lunch with another friend named Jenny and the topic of positive thinking and self-talk came up. I sat there with my mouth hanging open while they shared one story after another of improvements they were able to make in their lives by changing the way they were thinking.

"Jenny saw the look on my face and matter-of-factly said, 'It's not some weird kind of magic or something, Deanna. Everything you see around you right now started as a thought. The chair, the table, the way the signs are arranged. If we want to do something, we have to think about it first, and the more we think we can do it, the better chance that we will do it.' A light bulb went off in my head—a small one, like one of those little appliance bulbs that go in the oven, but it was a start. Later I asked Carla more about it and she said that even if I didn't believe the affirmations, just by saying them I was getting my mind to think something positive instead of thinking something negative. I figured it couldn't hurt me and decided to try it—mainly as an experiment. Carla told me I could take any of the affirmation cards around her house because she had them all memorized. I picked one on the refrigerator that said, 'I am strong enough to be gentle.' My kids often accused me of coming down too hard on them, so I thought, what the hell?

"I hid the card in my purse and I said the affirmation a few times a day when I saw it in there. After a week or so, I realized I was saying it to myself throughout the day, like when someone got in front of me in the grocery store line and when my son dropped the orange juice jug on the kitchen floor. I'm a little embarrassed to admit how well it worked. I was never a violent person, but I used to lose my temper and yell a lot. Now, when somebody pisses me off, that affirmation pops into my head, I take a deep breath and I am in control of my reaction."

in yourself. If the answer is yes, then circle it and put it on your "Things I Want to Change" list that you started back in chapter 3. If the "Ya, but" is just a knee-jerk reaction to not being comfortable with giving praise to yourself, draw a line through it and move on.

Discover the Beauty of Your Flaws

One of my favorite parables is about an elderly woman who had two large pots, each hung on opposite ends of a wooden pole that she carried across her shoulders to collect water from a stream and bring back to her home. One of the pots was perfect and always contained a full portion of water when the woman arrived home, but the other pot was cracked and would lose half of its water on the trip between the stream and the woman's house. The cracked pot was ashamed of its imperfection and felt miserable that it performed so poorly compared with its perfect counterpart. One day, the cracked pot could remain silent no longer and it spoke to the woman, lamenting its imperfection and apologizing for doing only half the work that the other pot did.

The old woman smiled and said to the pot, "What you think is a flaw is actually a blessing. The flowers that you see on your side of the path have grown because every day you water the seeds that I planted. I am able to enjoy these colorful flowers on my walk home every day and pick them to add beauty to our home." (This parable was passed on to me by a true friend who thought I needed to hear it.)

Instead of being embarrassed of your flaws, follow the example in this parable by starting to see how the parts of you that you consider flawed or imperfect are actually helping you move ahead personally and spiritually. Remember that what you think are flaws might also be helping other people to accept themselves. When I talk to others about my

HOT TIP
Step Up Your Plan

The day you reach your goal weight is the day to step up your plan, not the day to relax and take it easy. If you lost weight by walking a mile a day, step up your plan so that you're walking a mile and a half a day. You don't have to plan extra time into your workout or stay at the gym longer to do this. You can do it by adding extra steps to every part of your day.

My pedometer is one of the best investments that I've ever made. When I started on this journey, I could only walk a few steps at a time and now I can walk more than ten thousand. I don't make it to ten thousand each day by doing it all at once, though. I do it by taking steps all day long. The game is to use every free moment and every opportunity to make your steps add up. Every step counts, so count every step!

Instead of using the remote for your TV, get up and change the channel yourself. (Walking back and forth to the TV is much healthier than walking back and forth to the fridge!) When you're waiting for a bus or your carpool ride, pacing back and forth as fast as you can will rack up hundreds of steps. Walk a few blocks before hailing a cab and ask the driver to stop two or three blocks from where you're going. Make it a habit to get off the elevator a floor or two below the floor you're going to and walk down two to four flights of stairs before catching the elevator on the way down.

This will almost guarantee that you won't put pounds back on and can help you to drop more weight if that's one of your goals. Use every free moment to make your steps count. Little behavior changes like this have changed the way I think and transformed my life.

flaws, they can relate to me and are able to open up about their own lives and flaws, and that is an amazing connection that people can have and give to others. Numerous philosophers and psychologists have said that some of our greatest strengths can come out of what we consider our greatest weaknesses. For instance, it is by being afraid that we learn to start to see our courage. If we feel ashamed of our ignorance, we are motivated to learn more. If we think we take ourselves too seriously, we have a good reason to add more laughter to our lives. Instead of viewing the traits you don't like as flaws, why not see them as opportunities?

Darlene, a member of the Winners' Circle who lost thirty pounds and has kept it off for eight years, has a great story that shows how we never know how what we're doing is helping someone else. Even if we are like the cracked pot and think we are doing a poor job, chances are that someone is benefiting from our efforts. But the benefits are sometimes very different from what we think they should be. Darlene said she's always dreaded public speaking, even if it was just standing up in a meeting and saying her name and job title, or something as simple as that. She said when she has to present information to her colleagues, her face and neck turn beet red, and her voice shakes so much she can hardly control it.

Darlene said, "Speaking in public is one of my worst nightmares. I always feel like the people in the audience are putting me down in every possible way. I do everything I can to get out of those situations, but sometimes my boss makes me do it because he says I'm the only person in the office who can explain some of the material in a way that the other employees can understand it. I think he secretly believes that if I do it enough I'll get over my nervousness, but I doubt if that will ever happen. But something really sweet did happen one day and it gives me courage every time I have to present.

"One day, when I had to explain some new policy information to our staff, one of my coworkers had his ten-year-old daughter Amelia with him in the meeting. She had the day off from school so her dad brought her to work with him. She seemed very shy and never looked up at me when her dad introduced us. I struggled through my presentation, blushing, stammering, and sweating the entire time. When it was finally over, all I could think about was gathering my papers and getting out of the room as fast as I could. But as I was dashing for the door, Amelia was blocking my path. She looked me straight in the eyes and said, 'I want to thank you.' I couldn't imagine why she was thanking me. Nothing I said had anything to do with her and it probably didn't even make sense. 'You're welcome,' I said, 'but what are you thanking me for?' She said, 'The last two times I was supposed to do my book report, I told my teacher I felt sick and went to the nurse's office. I could tell you hated doing your report, but you did it anyway and my dad said you did a good job. I'm thanking you because the next time it's my turn to do my book report, I'm going to do it.'"

Stay Open to Possibilities

It's much more rewarding to start fresh every day when you practice staying open to promising possibilities. The better you get at living in the moment, the better chance you'll have of seeing possibilities and recognizing opportunities when they present themselves. It's normal to need some practice

HOW TO CREATE A PAPER TRAIL TO BETTER HEALTH

People who have lost a lot of weight, or who have skin that is less resilient because of their genetic makeup or their age, often suffer the effects of hanging skin. Dr. Elkwood says, "Aside from disliking the way it looks, skin folds can cause rashes, chafing, and back pain. It can also keep people from having a normal range of motion, which can hamper their ability to exercise."

One of the reasons gastric bypass surgery is covered by some insurance companies is that it helps people to lose weight so they can exercise and improve their cardiovascular health. If excess skin is stopping someone from being able to exercise (whether he or she had bypass surgery or not), that person is unable to improve his or her cardiovascular system. Excess skin can also be a constant negative reminder of the vestiges of the past and be a psychological barrier to living in the present.

Unfortunately, most insurance companies in this country consider the removal of excess skin cosmetic surgery rather than necessary surgery, and typically won't pay for it. I could not have a Pap smear because there was so much excess skin between my legs that the gynecologist couldn't perform the procedure. Despite this obvious health risk, insurance companies said that removing that excess skin was not necessary. They said it was cosmetic. Get real! I have received hundreds of requests from men and women asking me if I can help them to get financial assistance so they can afford to have the reconstructive surgery they need, and it breaks my heart.

According to Dr. Elkwood, "It is possible to create a paper trail documenting your health problems and medical issues to make a compelling case to your insurance company. There's no guarantee they will agree to pay for the surgery, but it's worth trying."

Dr. Elkwood says that each person who is insured has an individual contract with his or her insurance company that specifies whether or not certain forms of treatment and surgery are covered. Most companies have detailed criteria and want certain types of documentation before they will agree to cover the costs. In some cases, you can't know if the criteria are reached until after the surgery is done. For example, he explains, "Some companies will say that a certain amount of tissue must be removed in order to pay for a breast reduction. A surgeon can estimate how much tissue he or she is going to remove, but they can't know for sure until after the procedure is done."

He explains that there are often gray areas between what an insurance company considers reconstructive surgery and is willing to cover and what it considers cosmetic and is not willing to cover. For example, if someone lost twenty pounds and wants a tummy tuck, that's typically considered cosmetic. If someone lost two hundred pounds, that's more likely to be considered reconstructive and might be covered. But for the people who lost fifty pounds or a hundred pounds, the question is often up in the air. If you feel you need to have reconstructive surgery, Dr. Elkwood suggests that you try to build a case. He says, "Insurance companies look for things like back pain, inability to exercise, rashes, infections, boils, and things like that. If you're having these types of problems, it's important to document them."

If you're having rashes, make sure you see your medical doctor or dermatologist so there is a record. He says to ask your doctor to write a report summarizing your condition and what he or she feels needs to be done. It can be as simple as, "I've been treating John Doe over the past six months for rashes in the skin fold and feel he would benefit by having the excess skin removed." Dr. Elkwood says, "That's a lot more potent than you just telling the insurance company, 'I get rashes all the time.'" He also recommends that you photograph any visible problems caused by your excess skin and also suggests that you keep a diary of your symptoms and how they are treated. The record should include dates, the names of the physicians who treated you, a copy of prescriptions, and anything else that details what you are experiencing.

The key is to be as thorough with your documentation as possible and include as many experts and health care practitioners in your case as possible. If you can't ride the exercise bike because you have a skin fold that's in the way, have your personal trainer or the manager of your gym write a letter that says that. If you're having back pain, or other joint pains, see a chiropractor or internist and have them document it by writing a letter detailing the effects that your hanging skin is having on your posture and your spine, hips, knees, or other joints. If the hanging skin is causing chronic muscle stress, see a massage therapist and ask him or her to write a letter explaining how the hanging skin is causing you pain and other problems. The most important thing I can say about this is don't give up. If you need the surgery, explore every possible avenue until you find a way to get what you need done.

If you believe that insurance companies should cover reconstructive surgery for people who have lost a significant amount of weight, including excess skin removal, please write letters to your state's governor, senators, and representatives of Congress. See the resources section under "Weight Loss" for a Web site that provides names of government officials and contact information. This is very important. We must fight for ourselves!

in this area because many people are more programmed to anticipate bad things than good things.

Amy says, "It's a very common cognitive error that people make to predict negative outcomes for the future. It's called negative forecasting and people do it all the time." She says that to correct that cognitive error, you need to practice noticing when you're doing it, label the thought as negative forecasting, and remind yourself to stop it. People can engage in negative forecasting about something as trivial as not being able to find a parking space or as serious as predicting that something terrible is going to happen to them. I do this all the time and so do many people in my life.

She says, "People stir themselves up into a frenzy by anticipating what bad things are going to happen. But there's only one moment that you can live at a time. And so if you're negative forecasting about not getting a parking space, for example, you need to say to yourself, 'Okay, here I am in the moment. I'm not even in the parking lot yet. If there is no parking space, I will actually survive. It won't hurt me to have to walk farther. There are carts, so I'm not going to have to single-handedly lug twenty bags of groceries by myself.' The practice is about being mindful of the moment, noticing the thoughts you're having as they are going through your head and being able to label them in as nonjudgmental a way as you can." (Amy helped me to emotionally prepare for all the surgeries I've had. I used to worry for months in advance. Now I don't worry until the week of surgery. Hopefully, next time I won't worry until I'm getting wheeled into the operating room.)

Amy explains, "One of the biggest crimes we all commit is being very judgmental about everything. We criticize ourselves and other people so much that we limit our ability to stay open to possibilities without even realizing we're doing it. A lot of the time we're criticizing other people ahead of time so we can protect ourselves from feeling their criticism. This habit certainly isn't helping us to get where we want to be or create the relationships that we want to have. She says that to stay open, we must accept the reality of life by thinking, "Okay, right here in this moment, I'm doing this good thing, or I'm surviving this bad thing, but I need to avoid projecting into the future beyond the fact that I'm just going to enjoy or survive the moment that I'm in." She says, "The important thing is to remember that there's going to be another moment after this one. And if you're paying attention to where you are now then you're going to be more effective in the future. Focusing on the moment that you're in is more likely to make the future better than worrying about it will."

Another important part of being open to great things happening in your life is knowing that there is a balancing act between being spontaneous and staying in control. It's a fine line but it's one that is worth mastering. You must stay open to possibilities in order to learn new behaviors that can work for you. Once your game plan becomes a way of life, you can live in the moment without being out of control or going over the edge.

There is a really big difference between living *in* the moment and living *for* the moment. Living *in* the moment means being here now. Living *for* the moment means you are living just for that moment, as if that moment is the only one you will ever have. Doing that won't make your life better, but it might make your life worse, especially if you're not making choices based on the bigger picture of your life and everything and everyone who is most important to you. (Getting good at this has been a matter of maturing for me. And so what if I'm a late bloomer? At least I bloomed.)

BE AWARE OF YOUR RED FLAGS

The longer you maintain your weight, the better you'll get at reading the warning signs that tell you you're straying from your plan and need to get back on track. Everyone has different warning signs, but one thing that most red flags have in common is that you are doing something different from what's been working and you know (at least in the back of your mind) that you shouldn't be doing it!

Examples of Red Flags from the Winners' Circle

Red flags that let me know I might be heading for weight gain are . . .

Yvonne—The brightest red flag that I use as my rule of thumb is how my clothes fit. My face also gets puffy, and my hips start to spread.

Larry—Eating large portions of my favorite "snacks" that I am doling out to myself. Luckily, so far I have been able to catch myself before I gain.

Margaret—When I want to reach for food when I'm not physically hungry, it's a clue that something is going on with me emotionally and I need to deal with it instead of turning to food.

Deb—When I stopped counting the calories in "snack size" candy bars as though they simply didn't matter, it opened the door for absent eating of all my comfort foods. I thought as long as I didn't give up the exercise, I would negate all of the extra calories. Now I know better.

To Keep Your Love Life Fresh, Be Playful

When it comes to winning one day at a time with your love life, Dr. Greer says that one of the most important rules of thumb is to stay open to lighthearted sex play. She says, "Every sexual encounter doesn't have to be hot, serious, and steamy. Taking a more playful approach can make it easier and more comfortable to experiment, try new things, get to know each other's likes and dislikes, or get reacquainted, if you and your partner are taking sex off the back burner and putting it back on the top of your list."

To keep your sex life fresh and exciting, Dr. Greer suggests introducing two new scenarios to your repertoire. The first one can be summed up with one word. Spontaneity. She says, "Go for the moment. Be open to having sex *right here, right now,* instead of always waiting until the end of the day, or after you've had dinner or loaded the dishwasher. Flirt with your partner and make a pass as soon as he or she walks in the door. And the next time your lover gives you that special look or pinches your behind in a come-hither sort of way, drop everything and go for it."

The other scenario is the opposite of being spontaneous. In this case you plan to have sex, and make the preparation, buildup, and even the ending part of the action. She says, "You might spend the day e-mailing each other seductive messages and meet after work to shop for lingerie, scented candles, edible massage oil, or a new sex toy for the evening's adventure, all the while joking with each other, flirting, and using conversation and suggestive body language as a form of foreplay."

When the main event begins, she says, "Keep the playful theme going by touching each other with your hands and mouths, anywhere and everywhere but each other's erogenous zones. Now it's time to introduce games like show-and-tell, Simon says, master and slave, or anything playful that you both enjoy and feel comfortable playing. Some couples get into role-playing, but make sure that whatever you choose, you both want to do it and think it's fun. For a lot of couples part of the fun is laughing, giggling, calling each other silly pet names, and even acting young or using baby talk. Sex doesn't have to be serious and you don't always have to include gazing longingly into each other's eyes."

Dr. Greer stresses that the key is to be comfortable with each new thing you try, enjoy yourselves, and use some of these activities as a way to loosen up and expand your sexual horizons beyond the inhibitions that you may have. She says, "The afterplay can be giving each other massages or foot rubs, taking a bath or shower together, or just snuggling and holding each other close."

Define and Refine Your Style Sense

Now that you're a smaller size and have a new lifestyle, it's time to define and refine your style sense! Are you stuck in a fashion rut? Most people who are stuck in a rut of any kind don't know it, so before you answer no to that question, ask some trusted friends to give you their opinion about whether your wardrobe could use a little freshening up. You can also go to a store that offers personal shoppers at no extra charge, so explore the styles that they select for you. Try them on and see how similar or different they are from what's hanging in your closet. I know it can be hard to change the look you have had for years, but it is fun and very rewarding.

When you're going for a whole new look, one of the best ways to get an objective view of yourself in a variety of colors and styles is to have a friend take digital photos of you each time you step out of the dressing room. Instead of making decisions on the spot, take your time looking at the photos at home. Look at them the first time just to get a sense of how you think you look in each outfit. Then wait a week or so before you look at them again and see if your opinion has changed. Invite a couple close friends (who you know will be honest) to look at the photos and tell you which colors and styles they think are more flattering to your skin tone and figure. Once you've done all your research, it's time to buy! If you're on a tight budget, see if your favorite stores offer lay-away, or rank your top three to five favorites and buy one every month or so. (I used to have only four or five interchangeable outfits when I was fat, so my goal when I started to have clothing choices was to have thirty outfits, one for every day of the month without repeating. I've done more than well. In fact, it's time to ease up!) If you have a birthday coming up, don't be shy about letting your gift-buying friends and relatives know that you have some fabulous clothes on your wish list. I've always thought that clothing stores should offer gift registries for people who have dropped a few sizes and are in need of a new wardrobe, but so far no one's capitalized on that idea.

Avoid Fashion Faux Pas!

After carrying around extra weight for months, years, or in my case, decades, it's very tempting to want to go clothing crazy and show off your new size with total abandon. Do yourself a huge favor and resist that urge! Of course you want to wear styles and fashions that highlight your best features and celebrate your new lifestyle, but you can't make up for lost time and trying to recapture your younger days by shopping in the junior department is definitely a no-no! Another fashion faux pas to avoid is exposing too many parts of yourself at one time. Put together outfits that draw attention to only one of your qualities at a time. If you're wearing a short skirt to show off your legs, don't wear a plunging neckline too. If your décolletage is accenting your breasts, don't wear a midriff or short shorts at the same time. Sometimes the sexiest and most seductive thing you can do is to expose skin that is not typically thought of as sexual, such as by wearing a top that exposes your shoulders or long sleeves that are slit to show a hint of the skin on your arms. Sweaters and dresses with Vs in the back and long skirts with slits that go just a little above the knee are all great ways to flash a hint of skin while looking classy, instead of slutty. And as my mom always tells me, "You don't have to wear everything in your jewelry box all at once." And please remember, while it's okay to get others' opinions of what you should wear, don't give up your personal sense of style. That's what makes you unique.

Don't Fall for Trends, But Do Try Variety!

Don't fall for trends, but be open to incorporating a variety of styles into your wardrobe so you can dress the way you feel, or present the image that shows off your personality whether you're going on a date, being interviewed for a potential job, or attending your class reunion. Don't wear a blazer every day if you want to look sexy! And don't dress like a sex kitten at work if you want your business associates to take you seriously. One of the most creative and fun ways to put an original outfit together is to mix and match different styles. If you've never paid much attention to fashion or style but you want to have fun with them now, buy a few magazines and cut out the photos of the looks you like. You can even put them up inside your closet door or on a bulletin board in your bedroom as a guideline for what types of pieces and accessories go well together.

The key is to have fun, take chances, and try new things. Go out of your way to try on clothes, hats, sunglasses, and shoes that are absolutely not what you would typically wear. Just because you're used to wearing a certain style doesn't mean that it shows off your best features. Fashion make-overs are a lot of fun and sometimes stunning because most people don't wear the styles and cuts of clothing that make them look their best. Take a friend along to a few stores that you never shop in and ask him or her to randomly pull items off the rack for you to try on. I never thought I'd look good in off-the-shoulder blouses, but now I love them! Not only do they make me feel feminine, but even when I'm bloated I can count on my shoulders looking good!

That Old Black Ain't No Magic at All!

Does your closet have so much black in it that it looks like you're mourning? Many people, particularly women who have been heavy, seem to have a hard time separating themselves from their basic black wardrobe. For years, every article of clothing I owned was black. My life took an exciting turn the day I finally discovered that old black ain't magic! I never liked uniforms, but I might as well have had one, since every day was a repeat of the day before—long black stretch pants and a black top with three-quarter-length sleeves.

I was living in a hospital eating disorder unit in Biloxi, Mississippi, and one hot, humid day in July our group was outside taking our daily walk. I was trudging along in my uniform, wondering if I had ever been any hotter or more uncomfortable in my life and wondering why in the hell these eating disorder programs always seemed to be in the South, when one of the people in the group asked me, "Why are you wearing black in this heat?" What could I say? "Pardon me, but haven't you noticed that I'm fat?" I honestly didn't know that wearing black in the sun made you feel hotter. I'd worn it for years, rain or shine.

Later that day I shared with the group that I felt like I looked too fat in any color other than black. My therapist said, "Why don't you get just one shirt in a different color, wear it for our group, and we'll tell you the truth about whether the black shirt makes you look any thinner or not." I agreed to call my seamstress in New York and order a beige top. That was as much color as I could handle!

I also had no idea that I was in a rut by wearing black every day, but then most people who are in a fashion rut don't know it and that's why they keep wearing the same things day in, day out. Sometimes other people's honest feedback can be like a magic mirror. It can show you the truth that you don't see when you look into your own mirror!

Two weeks later I was standing in front of the group in my beige top. I *did* feel cooler. One by one these people whom I had come to trust assured me that I looked great and not even a pound heavier. The next top I ordered was magenta, then lavender, jade, sky blue, and eventually I had every color in the rainbow. I discovered that I loved the world in color! I even ordered colored pants. I started with navy (be reasonable!). I wear black now once in a while to look sexy, but never because I think it makes me look thinner!

So add some color to your world! Try on clothes in all "color seasons" and decide what looks best. Wearing colors can make you feel more cheerful and look younger. Find out how you look and feel in every color. When you first see yourself in the dressing room mirror wearing a new color, your impression might be negative, just because it's something you're not used to. If you don't have a friendly photographer with you, at least give yourself a few minutes of wearing the color before you rule it out.

Downsize Your Wardrobe Gradually

Whether you've lost twenty pounds or hundreds, the questions of if and when to get rid of your clothes in bigger sizes eventually come up. Ridding yourself of the old clothes is as important as ridding yourself of the pounds. But don't get rid of them all at once or you'll either have to buy an entire wardrobe or join a nudist colony! Seriously, if you hold on to all your old clothes, you are reinforcing the fear that you are not going to maintain your new size. On the other hand, if you get rid of everything immediately, it can make you feel so pressured about the keeping the weight off that you can create a state of panic for yourself.

Based on my experience and the experience of people in the Winners' Circle, the best approach is to shed your old clothes the same way you shed your pounds—gradually. Each time you buy something new, give away something from your old wardrobe. If you buy two new things, give away two old things. By doing this, you can slowly transform your closet in a way that doesn't feel traumatic or scary.

Keep a few articles of clothing from when you were your heaviest because seeing those clothes next to the ones you fit in now is very rewarding. Every time I hold up my old red bloomers I can hardly believe I used to wear panties that are big enough to be a country's flag!

Follow the Five-Year Rule

Have you ever noticed that some people never change their look? Some even have the same hairstyle they had in high school. Others have wardrobes that don't include anything that was ever in style. Now, don't get me wrong. I have never been a follower of the latest trend. For me, fashion sense is all about wearing what we love, whether it's "in fashion" or not. Follow the Five-Year Rule, and make at least one small change in your look every five years. A few simple changes can make you look younger and fresher and keep you from sliding into a fashion rut. As you evaluate your wardrobe, keep in mind that sometimes just one or two accessories can take an outfit you bought ten years ago and bring it right up to date. Adding the right accessories can work wonders for your wardrobe, and it's a lot cheaper than buying a whole new outfit.

In addition to keeping your closet current, consider making at least a slight change in your hairstyle. If you've had a middle part for years, try a side part. If you've always had a blunt cut, consider having your stylist cut in a few layers. Making a dramatic change in your hairstyle can be really fun, and many women and men swear by it because they say it makes them feel so much better about themselves. But if the idea of making a big change seems too scary, start with a few subtle highlights, or a slightly more vibrant color. If your hair is long, consider having a few inches taken off to make it healthier and give it more volume. If you really want to be versatile and have fun with different looks, buy a couple wigs! The simple changing of a hairstyle makes you look instantly more youthful. Eventually, the Farrah Fawcett feathers will come back, but for now ease up!

The other change that many women fail to make is to keep their makeup up to date. Your skin tone and resiliency changes over time and simple changes like switching from a pressed to a loose powder can make a big difference. Try a new blush, a softer eye shadow, and experiment with a few different-colored eyeliners and lip colors. Remember that just like when you're branching out to wear different styles and colors of clothing, your first reaction to a new type of makeup might be negative just because you're so used to the way you've looked for years.

At the very least, take advantage of the free makeovers that many department stores and cosmetic counters offer. To be able to accurately assess whether you like it or not, leave the makeup the way the stylist does it for the rest of the day. Every hour or so, take a look in the mirror and see how your opinion changes. By the end of the day, you still may not like the dark eyeliner or shiny lip gloss, but you may decide that the new shade of blush or eye shadow is actually perfect for you.

ONE PURCHASE, THREE PURPOSES

Makeup doesn't have to cost a fortune or take hours to apply. Buy a blush in an earth tone that complements you. (Nothing too pink because that won't look good on your eyes.) Take a blush brush and sweep the blush over your whole eyelid and crease of your eye. Blend it well. Then use the same blush for your cheeks, and finally, take your index finger and tap the blush onto your lips as lipstick. It will feel dry, but you can take care of that by applying a clear lip gloss on top. If you have a few seconds more, add mascara, and finito, you're done. You will look prettier in minutes. Being on top of your beauty game is sure to boost your self-esteem!

THE IMPERFECT TEN

The Top Ten Ways to Start Your Day Fresh and Finish Strong

1. Pace yourself. Don't rush around in a tizzy to get dressed and get out the door. Get up a bit earlier and give yourself enough time to reaffirm the plans you made last night for today.

2. Decide what is the maximum you are willing to do and then decide what is the minimum you can accomplish that day and still feel good about yourself.

3. Make sure at least one of your goals for the day moves you in the direction of your biggest dream, even if it's one phone call to set something in motion.

4. You must have breakfast. If you don't, then look at it as a clear warning sign of danger ahead!

5. Decide when (not if!) you will exercise or do some other physical activity during the day, even if it's only a brisk walk.

6. Make a connection by phone, via e-mail, or in person with one person who has a very positive effect on you.

7. Before you leave the house remember to defrost something for dinner or make a dinner plan so you're not caught off guard at that vulnerable time at the end of the day when you arrive home tired and hungry.

8. Take time to decompress from your day (whatever that means to you). For me, it's walking my dog to the outdoor Starbucks to have an iced coffee, chill out, and put things in perspective.

9. Always have low-calorie finger foods ready in the fridge.

10. Have a nighttime ritual to wrap up your day. I sometimes make a pot of decaf tea and think of all the good I did today and what I need to work on tomorrow. It's at this time that I clean the day's slate. If I overate, that's the time that I "erase" it and decide to start fresh tomorrow.

STEP 7

Feed Your Hopes and Dreams
Make Every Day Count

Hold fast to your dreams, for if dreams die
life is a broken-winged bird that cannot fly.
Hold fast to dreams, for if dreams go
life is a barren field frozen with snow.

—Langston Hughes, poet and novelist

When I was at my heaviest and my mother, who I had been living with in New York, decided to move to Florida, most of my relatives and friends assumed that I'd go with her. At that point in my life it was very hard for me to get around by myself, so when I announced that I wasn't going to Florida, I was going to rent an apartment in Brooklyn, I surprised a lot of people. What I didn't tell them was that in my heart I knew that if I was going to have a chance at my dream to be a working actress and published author, I had to stay close to New York. Shortly after that move, I landed a film role, and now you are reading my book. When it comes to hopes

226

and dreams, sometimes we have to be willing to take a leap of faith.

My dreams to be an actress and published author helped carry me through the darkest days of my life. Today, the same dreams inspire me, keep me focused, and help me to stick with my winning game plan. My hopes and dreams give me strength during the challenging times that I now know are part of life, no matter how much or how little we weigh.

Step 7 shows you how your hopes and dreams can help you stick with your game plan and stay in the Winners' Circle forever! You are about to learn how to get in touch with your dreams, bring them to life, and share them with the people you care about. In this chapter, you'll also find out why it's so important to reach beyond yourself and how doing that can support your commitment to maintain your weight. Since so many people who are single are looking for someone to share their life and their dreams with (including me!), this chapter also gives you some ideas for how to go about finding the right person for you. (And if he's great but not right for you, please pass him along to me!)

Keeping your hopes and dreams alive and taking one step after another to make them come true will make you feel energized, motivated, and excited about life. Knowing that it's up to you to create the future that you dream about is thrilling and sometimes a little scary. But when you feel scared, sad, or anxious, practice feeding your hopes and dreams instead of feeding yourself. (I figure that if I feed my dreams as much as I used to feed myself, my success is practically guaranteed!)

Feeding Your Dreams Makes You Feel Full

As we've said, once the compliments die down and the thrill of fitting into smaller-size clothes wears off, and you are facing challenges, struggling with problems, and dealing with the ups and downs of everyday life, you may discover (probably to your horror) that your motivation to maintain your weight is sliding. Very few people believe that this is going to happen. Most people, especially in the first few months or year after reaching their goal weight, will swear on a stack of takeout menus that being smaller is—in itself—enough motivation to stay that way. Okay, pay close attention. I want you to imagine the obnoxious sound of one of those game show buzzers that means, "Wrong!" If the answer was right, then most of the people who lose weight would keep it off, instead of putting it back on. So please don't start kidding yourself after you've made it this far. Yes, it's possible that you are the exception to the rule, but why take chances when you can take precautions instead?

The cold, hard, ugly truth is that your maintenance game plan is only as good as your commitment. And when your motivation starts to slip and slide, it's very easy to let the daily grind crush your determination to stay healthy and fit. (There's a reason it's called the daily grind!) So if you want to have a lifelong reason to stay in the game, keep the weight off, and live the most fulfilling life that's possible for you, you need to get in touch with your most heartfelt hopes and dreams.

For example, Margaret, an artist who is in the Winners' Circle, says that since she lost weight, part of her passion is to help other people improve the quality of their lives. She says, "I have never been more fit, healthy, or happy in my life. My life has been profoundly changed with what I learned during my weight loss journey. Not only did my relationship with food change, but also the way I approach life's problems and challenges. My self-esteem skyrocketed as my self-image changed from one that was very negative to one of self-acceptance and love." She says she didn't used to exercise much at all and she rarely wanted to go out. "I used to be shy and distanced myself socially."

Now she and her husband are taking ballroom dancing lessons, she runs about thirty miles a week, and she does aerobics and trains with weights twice a week. She says, "I love being active now, and even on days when I'm not feeling very energetic, I at least do some yoga. And I usually find out that the energy I need to run is there after all!"

Margaret says, "My purpose is to be a loving presence with myself and other people." She is also inspired to keep using her creativity with her artwork and to be a guide and a mentor for others. She says that on difficult days, her dreams and her purpose keep her going.

We all have at least one or two things that we would love to do or be, so if your mind just played a little trick on you by thinking, "I don't have any hopes or dreams," don't believe it for a second! Have you ever asked little kids what they want to be when they grow up and had them say, "Nothing"?

Of course not. When kids are bright-eyed and excited about life, they want to be firefighters, doctors, teachers, plumbers, dancers, astronauts, writers, airplane pilots, and all sorts of other things. Lots of kids will rattle off a whole list of things they want to be. It's not until they get older and enough people tell them they can't live their dreams that they give them up, lock them away in the depths of their hearts, and forget about them. So there is definitely something that you would love to do; you just have to help that "something" to rise to the surface again.

Yvonne, a member of the Winners' Circle for about two years, says she always had a dream of being an athlete and a model. She says, "But I was always fat and dowdy and the other kids at school taunted me." She said as her fortieth birthday approached, she decided enough was enough and committed to doing whatever she had to do to lose the extra forty pounds she was carrying and keep it off for good. She's already been in a national commercial for Jenny Craig, and since running is her hobby, she says she'd love to pose for a sports magazine.

Ben, a member of the Winners' Circle for more than five years, said ever since he was a little boy he wanted to be a firefighter like his dad and his uncle. But he was overweight as a child and by the time he was in high school he was obese. He said, "I still had the dream of being a firefighter, but I could barely get around myself, let alone carry the heavy hoses or move fast. So I decided I'd better find a job that didn't take so much out of me and I became an accountant. I have a great job and like what I do, but after I lost weight, the idea of being a fireman kept popping into my head. After a few months, I stopped at the local fire station and asked what I had to do to be a volunteer. When I found out that if I took a few classes, did some training exercises, and passed the test, I could be part of the volunteer squad; I was like a little kid again. I've been a volunteer now for a couple of years and I love it. There's nothing like the feeling I get when I know I'm helping to save somebody's house or business. I've even rescued a couple of kittens that were afraid to come down out of trees—just like in the movies!"

Sometimes Dreams Change

Even though a lot of people like Yvonne and Ben still have the same dreams they had when they were younger, a lot of people have different dreams or have added new dreams to their list of old ones. You might have also had a long-held dream that you realized wasn't right for you and have since let go. Or maybe you still have an old dream in mind, but it no longer gives you the same kind of joy or excitement as it used to. You also could be holding on to (or living) a dream that was actually someone else's dream for you, but that doesn't feel right to you now or, worse yet, feels like a burden. One way to give your dreams a test run is to close your eyes and imagine yourself living a day in the life of your dream. Try to see the details in living color. What are you doing? How do you feel? Are you smiling? Does your heart feel like it could do a song-and-dance routine? If not, it might be time to let go of that dream and do a little soul-searching to get in touch with what you'd really love to do. Then be willing to pay the price to go for it. It won't be easy, but it will be worth it. (Take that leap of faith!)

For example, Belinda, who has maintained her weight loss for six years, went back to college when she was fifty-three to get a degree in psychology and then went another two years to get her master's degree. Today, at the age of fifty-nine, she is a social worker and loves it. She said, "I liked accounting when I got into it, but over the years I discovered that I was spending more time counseling people on their personal lives than on their finances. I realized that helping people to make better choices was what I liked most about my job and every year doing taxes and reviewing financial portfolios got more and more boring. I could have kept doing it and found other ways to help people through volunteering or being a mentor, but I thought it would be invigorating to go back to college and be surrounded by all those young minds. My friends thought I was crazy and it was hard to get back into the discipline of studying, doing homework, and writing papers, but it was also thrilling. I love what I'm doing now and I feel more alive than I have in decades!"

If you don't know what your dream is, don't worry; you'll have a chance to start figuring that out in a few minutes. In the meantime, it might help if you consider that human beings, by our very nature, have a desire to improve our circumstances and lot in life. We don't sit around daydreaming about making our lives worse. We think about what it would be like if things were better. For example, I'd bet that no one wakes up in the morning and says, "I wish I wasn't so smart," or "I wish I had less money," or "I wish I wasn't so generous or helpful." I'm pretty sure I've never met anyone who wishes that more people were starving and homeless or that the planet was more polluted. Wanting to improve ourselves, our circumstances, and the world in which we live (or at least our little corner of it) seems like part of human nature. If you're not doing that, or know other people who aren't doing that, it's probably not because the desire isn't there. There are thousands of different reasons (a.k.a. excuses) that people don't do the things they want to do, but none of them have to do with a lack of desire. So just accept that you have a natural desire to improve your life, your circumstances, and maybe even the world by pursuing a heartfelt dream. And you might just have a mission or a purpose, so don't rule that out. Accepting that reality will make it a hell of a lot easier for you to get in touch with your hopes and dreams (if you don't already know what they are) and actually start living them.

Bring Your Dreams to Life

There is absolutely no good reason why you can't start pursuing your hopes and dreams in some way, shape, or form right now. I started writing this book long before I ever knew when or even if anyone would want to publish it. (Once in a twelve-step program meeting, I heard someone say, "Fake it till you make it," and that is what I've been doing my whole life. I faked my belief in myself until it actually became real.) If you stop yourself from going after your dreams until you can see that you will achieve them, you'll never get started because there are no guarantees in life except that it will end someday. If your dream is to be a best-selling author, you can start writing a book today and achieve something important, whether or not the book becomes a best-seller or ever gets published at all. The act of writing the book will open many doors and you will learn so much about yourself. (Trust me!) Artists don't wait to paint until they are guaranteed to sell. They paint for the beauty in the way that it makes them feel. On that merit alone, it's a good enough reason to pursue your dreams. Was I not an actress before I was paid to do a movie? Of course I was. I was an actress from the moment I was in my first production of *You're a Good Man, Charlie Brown* at age ten at my family's beach club. If your dream is to be an actor, go for it. Audition for a local play, take acting classes, or start your own community theater. Whether your name ever ends up in lights is not even half as important as doing what you love and using your abilities and talents. You may not be able to solve the world's hunger problem, but you can organize and participate in efforts to feed the hungry in your own backyard. The secret to being inspired about life every day is making a difference by doing what you love to do in whatever way you are able to do it. That's also one of the best ways to contribute something meaningful to your family, friends, and community. I once heard someone say that at the end of our lives, the question God will ask us is, "Have you used everything that I gave you?"

Dr. Nadler has been guiding people through the process of getting in touch with their life dreams and taking the action steps to live those dreams for more than fifteen years, so you're in for a mind-shifting, heart-opening experience. And by the way, as the aliens like to say in old movies, "Resistance is futile," so do what she says.

Define Your Dream

So what is your dream? Not just the dream for your body but the dream for your life. Take out your Winners' Circle Workbook and begin a new section called "Hopes and Dreams." The best way to really know for sure what your hopes and dreams are is to begin to listen and get to know that one true voice in your head—it knows what it's talking about, so trust it. Dr. Nadler says, "This generally means learning how to discern 'who' is speaking. It can be a challenge to distinguish which 'voice' is actually *your* voice and which voices are repeating the ideas or beliefs of someone else who is or was in your life. The key is to separate your true hopes and dreams from what other people want for you."

A really great way to tune in to knowing exactly what your hopes and dreams are is to take a little trip down memory lane. Okay, I know we all know it's not a good thing to dwell on the past, but in this case it's okay, I promise. Close your eyes and remind yourself of all the things you loved to do when you were a kid. (For me, I loved to ice skate, make jewelry, and entertain groups of people by having plays in the neighborhood backyards.) Make a list of these things in your workbook and then add the new loves that you have discovered over the years. Remembering what you loved in the past and adding the new things can help you to discover what your passion is now. Dr. Nadler says to pick one of the things you love, get comfortable, and close your eyes. Picture yourself doing that activity from start to finish. Leave out no details. By the end of this exercise you will have a very good idea of how doing something you love makes you feel. She says, "You might feel your heart beating faster or your fingers tingling or a sense of heat in your body." (When I do this I get all excited and I usually get up and start making some sort of plan; it's amazing how this works.)

The way I know that something is right for me is that it feels the same way as it does when I fall in love. When I write, act, or motivate people, and especially when I make someone have a belly laugh, I literally experience my heart racing, I want to cry happy tears of accomplishment, and I sometimes get the butterflies I had when I first fell in love. This is my voice! The voices that are not mine are the voices that say, "You're too old to start that now," or "You're too old to have a good chance to find a mate." Those are not my voices!

Once you are in touch with how you feel when you are in a state of joy, you are ready to do the next part of the exercise. Dr. Nadler says to close your eyes again and imagine that there is a door right in front of you and that your hopes and dreams are on the other side of that door. Put your hand on the doorknob and ask yourself the million-dollar question: "What would I truly love in my life?" Then open the door, look around, and write about what you see. Just putting those words on paper will start to make your dream feel possible and real.

Dr. Nadler explains, "You may have to repeat this exercise a few times before you can get a clear image. Sometimes the images might not make sense and the first time or so that you do this exercise, you may not see anything at all. Don't give up! One day—probably sooner than you think—you will open the door and 'Wow!' it will all be perfectly clear and you will know that these hopes and dreams are truly from your heart."

Write It Down

Writing your hopes and dreams down helps you to add important details so instead of having a foggy idea, you have a crystal-clear picture of what you want.

Dr. Nadler says, "It is important to recognize that your life is not only your body and your physical health but also your relationships, career, finances, family, mental health, and spirituality. In looking at your dreams, consider all the areas of your life and see how staying healthy and fit will affect each one."

Find the most comfy, cozy place in your home and use that as your quiet space to spend an hour or so answering the following burning questions.

How will maintaining my goal weight benefit my:
Health?
Career or job?
Financial security or freedom?
Relationships (significant other, children, relatives,
    friends)?
Mental health?
Spirituality?

Write as many answers to each of those questions as you feel are important. You may not have clear answers for all the questions yet, but do your best to come up with at least a couple answers for each.

Next, Dr. Nadler says to ask yourself, "If I could do, be, and have whatever I want in all areas of my life and knew that my hopes and dreams were truly meant for me to live, what would my life be like?" Write whatever is in your heart. Don't spare any of the details. Spell this out exactly the way you would want it to be in a perfect world. Begin by writing, "My deepest hopes and dreams are . . ." Continue writing until you have covered all the juicy details that make you feel alive and that would make you excited about getting up each day.

Once you have it all written down, review what you wrote and circle or use a highlighter to identify the things that make you smile and give you a true sense of joy. Use the information you have circled or highlighted to write a summary statement (or purpose statement) that captures the essence and all the important details of your hopes and dreams. Begin your statement by writing:

I [your name] am willing to pursue the following hopes and dreams and make them real in my life:

Make a photocopy of your summary statement that you can carry with you in your wallet or purse. Some people have their summary statements written in calligraphy and framed; others put them on their bulletin board or in other places around their home. You can even use your summary or purpose statement as your computer screen saver. The idea is to read it at least once a day.

Dr. Nadler says, "Sometimes when people look at their dreams for the future, they seem so big that they can be paralyzing instead of motivating. By taking a big dream and turning it into small steps, you make it manageable and it's easier for you to wrap your mind around the idea that you can truly do what it is you're dreaming about."

Now comes the part that you have to be brutally honest with yourself about. Ask yourself, "What am I honestly willing to do to make my hopes and dreams reality?" Write the first three action steps you are willing to take in your workbook and then schedule them in your date book or calendar. When you have completed those steps, schedule the next three steps. Add new steps to your list as you discover them. (Every single day I do at least one thing that will move me toward my big dreams. It could be as simple as making a phone call to set the actions in motion.)

Reaching Beyond Yourself

The idea of reaching beyond yourself is to give your attention to projects and activities that take your mind off your problems or personal drama. But reaching beyond yourself can also be a way to figure out or remember your hopes and dreams. If you still aren't sure about what you most want to do or be, do some research on people who you admire. Think of three or four people you know who are happy and successful and then find out more about them. What, if anything, do they have in common with each other? (I've been doing this my whole life—studying people who are able to keep their weight off.) What do they do that you think you'd like to do? What is it about their lifestyle, career, or personality that you find most appealing? If they are friends or family members, call them up, let them know what you're doing, and set up a time to meet with them. If they are acquaintances or colleagues, ask them if they can make some time for you to have a talk with them. Tell them you admire them and explain that you are exploring some options for your future. Since you are impressed with them and what they're doing, you'd like to know more about them. Most people will be flattered beyond belief and some might even volunteer to be your mentor. Be sure to ask them how they knew they wanted to do what they're doing with their life and why it means so much to them.

It's important to get in touch with your hopes and dreams because they can keep you going during times when not much else can. Not only do they add meaning to your life,

but they also help to keep you out of trouble by giving you productive things to do. When I am engaged in something I love doing, food is not on my mind! When I first lost weight and didn't have something important to focus on, I managed to get into all sorts of mischief. If you're smiling or laughing right now, you know exactly what I'm talking about!

Having hopes and dreams also keeps you from getting the "So What?" syndrome that so many people seem to have. Symptoms of this syndrome include feelings of boredom, lack of curiosity, and just feeling tired. People with "So What?" syndrome have very little meaning or purpose in their lives. People suffering with this might often wonder, "Is this all there is to my life?"

Honestly, I can hardly comprehend that way of living. Even if you haven't figured out what your hopes and dreams are, life itself is so stimulating and exciting that I just don't get how people can be bored. There are so many things I want to do and so many places I want to see that there is never enough time in a day. I used to feel like I lost years of my life, but now I'm beginning to understand that the years I spent isolating myself have helped me to truly appreciate every minute that I have left.

Focusing on Others

Another important part of reaching beyond yourself is reaching out to help other people. Amy says, "If you find yourself sitting around ruminating about your struggles, it's

a sure sign that you need to focus on someone else. Turning your attention to helping other people who might be less fortunate than you can shift your attention, change your emotional state, and make you feel more connected to the world and less burdened by your own issues. It can also be a great way to remind yourself of the things in your life that you have to be grateful for. There are lots of ways you can help others. Just look around you. Consider volunteering for a community project or a social service organization."

When you start to get into the practice of focusing on others, all sorts of ideas will pop into your mind. There are hundreds of ways to do something nice for someone else. My family and friends have always been very generous to me. They gave me jewelry, makeup, music, and pretty things for my apartment. When I was out of money, someone would show up and take me out to dinner or bring takeout dinners. When I lost my own car, my friend Timmy bought a used car for us to share. My friend Teena and her husband used to bring bags full of groceries.

But I don't think my friends ever knew I was generous because I used to feel like I had to hoard things for myself. (Hoarding is a common addict behavior.) Now I love giving things to other people. It's one of the biggest thrills of my life. It's the most unreal thing to find out I have this quality that I didn't know I had! It was there all along, but it was buried. Several people in the Winners' Circle said they used to hoard possessions, just like they did food. Carmella said, "I used to buy other people birthday gifts and end up keeping

them for myself. I couldn't seem to part with anything I liked and couldn't even give away some of the things I didn't like. I gave gift certificates to friends and family members for years because I would always have some reason why I had to keep the present that I originally bought for them."

Roxanne said she was a hoarder for years. She said, "I had an entire basement stuffed with things I bought at flea markets and garage sales. I had so much stuff that I had to buy thirty-two shelves, the tall kind that go the whole way up to my ceiling, just to fit it all in there. I had no idea what I was going to do with all of it. To tell you the truth, I didn't even know what all was down there. After I lost weight and started seeing a shrink, I started to understand that I was doing the same thing with junk as I used to do with food. I used to think spending fifty dollars on a nice dinner was crazy, but I didn't think there was anything wrong with spending fifty dollars on a grocery cart full of junk food. I was at my goal weight for almost three years before I felt like I could part with what I started to call my basement fat. I still have a few shelves full of the things I really like, but the rest of it I sold at a garage sale or gave away."

But there are also people in the Winners' Circle who had the opposite problem when they were overweight—they couldn't stop giving things to other people. George said, "I was a chronic people pleaser. I felt like the only way I could make people happy and keep them liking me was to give them things. Every time I shopped I'd come home with four or five things for other people. I'm just lucky I found a good therapist and was able to stop doing that before I got cable, because those shopping channels would have put me into bankruptcy!" (Amen, brother!)

Alice said, "I was a chronic gift giver and after I lost weight that habit got worse for a couple of years!" She says she still has to fight the urge to give people things as a way to win their approval. She said, "Even though I understand that people are my friends because they like me, it's still sometimes hard to believe that they really like me just for who I am. When I think I upset someone or disappointed them, the first thought that comes to mind is, 'What can I give them?' I can usually stop myself from going through with it now, but I still go hog wild for birthdays and weddings."

A lot of the people in the Winners' Circle are into random acts of kindness and say that when they start to feel sorry for themselves, they can change their mood by doing something nice for someone else, even if it's something very small. (For me, giving all my expensive fat clothes away was a thrill! I brought them to a local eating disorder hospital in my area and anonymously dropped them off. I laughed once when I went to visit a good friend in that hospital and saw a stranger wearing my size 60 leopard robe that I had made.)

Anne said, "I had just ordered a salad at a fast-food drive-thru and was sitting in line smelling the French fries and feeling sort of deprived, when I noticed this old man walking along the curb a few cars behind me picking up change. I grabbed my wallet and discreetly dropped all the change

I had—at least a few dollars' worth—onto the curb. As I was driving away, I saw the guy picking up the change with a huge smile on his face. He looked like he just won the lottery. It was great!"

Random Acts of Kindness from the Winners' Circle
Put nickels or dimes in the coin return slots of pay
    phones or candy machines.
Give someone a sincere compliment.
If you notice that a parking meter is about to expire,
    buy the person a little extra time by inserting some
    change.
Buy a helium balloon and give it to the next parent with
    a small child that you see.
Pay the toll of the person behind you at the tollbooth.
Give your take-home bag of leftovers to a homeless
    person.
Offer someone your seat on the bus or train.
Double the next tip you give.
Shovel the snow from your neighbor's sidewalk.
Take care of a friend's or relative's children for an
    evening.

Finding the Mate of Your Dreams

Okay, here we go. I knew I'd eventually have to cover this. Most of the single men and women I know would really like to find a mate. There's no doubt that finding the right man or woman to share your life with is tricky, no matter who you are or what you look like. But people who have struggled with their weight often have an even harder time than others because they usually have self-esteem issues. These people are sometimes so self-conscious or worried about pleasing the people they date that they hardly notice whether they really like the person they're on a date with. In the most extreme cases, every date can turn into a "How do I make him or her fall madly in love with me?" challenge before they even know if the person they are trying to sweep off his or her feet is someone who is really worth sweeping.

On the opposite side of the fence, you might have unrealistic fantasies or expectations that can only be fulfilled in fairy tales, romance novels, or made-for-TV movies. I'm not saying you shouldn't go for what you want, I'm just saying that it's a good idea to do a reality check to make sure what you're looking for is possible. (I scared several men off in the beginning with my unrealistic fantasies about romance and all that it entails.)

Dr. Greer explains, "Very often when people think of their dream guy or dream gal, they think of all the qualities that they want in a partner, but they don't think about the interaction between their dream mate and themselves. For example, a lot of people have a list of traits they want their partner to have. A woman might say, 'I'm looking for a man who's tall, smart, attractive, and has a good sense of humor.' It's okay to want all of those things, but it makes more sense to first think about the interaction that you want to have with someone and then define their individual traits. For example: Does he or she ask questions about you? Does he/she listen to you without interrupting? Do you laugh a lot together? Do you feel 'at home' with him or her? Do you feel like he/she gets you? By being clear about the interactional component first, you are creating a better search engine. It increases your chances of finding someone who is right for you and decreases the odds of dismissing someone (based on your list of desired traits) who could be perfect for you before you really get to know them."

So take out your Winners' Circle Workbook and write a description of the relationship you want to have with your dream mate. Dr. Greer says, "It's important to have some things in common, but it's even more important that you're both open to expanding your horizons, learning, growing, and participating in what each other enjoys. You might write something like, 'We will treat each other with respect, be accountable, and keep our word to one another. We will both like going out to eat, watching funny movies, and traveling. We will be affectionate with each other and be lighthearted enough to laugh about our minor difficulties and differences and mature enough to talk through our problems.'"

Next, she says that you should write down how you want to feel when you're with your dream mate. She says, "You might say you want to feel safe, secure, desirable, self-confident, comfortable, appreciated, validated, or acknowledged. Just write down the sentence, 'When we're together I want to feel . . .' and finish that sentence with whatever is true for you. You can make your description as long or short as you want, as long as you have a clear picture of what the two of you will be like together." You can also write down couples, either whom you know or who are famous, that you consider role models for the type of relationship you are looking for.

Dr. Greer says, "Once you have the most important part of your search plan in place, you can write down the specific traits you imagine your dream mate having. Do you find a particular body type more appealing than other types? Are you looking for an extrovert or an introvert? Your goal with this part of the plan is to be as specific as you can be, while being willing to keep an open mind."

KNOW YOUR TRIGGERS

If you know what weakens your will to win the maintenance game or triggers your temptation to overeat, skip your workout, or do anything else that can sabotage your success, you can take steps—ahead of time—to protect yourself. Take out your Winners' Circle Workbook and make a list of your triggers. Next to each one, write down what you can do to keep that trigger from setting you up for a fall.

Winners' Circle Triggers

Donna—Primarily emotional situations, stress, being lonely, homesick, or depressed.

Yvonne—Eating out of entitlement. If I survived a hard day at work, I could feel that I deserve something greasy, salty, doughy, or sweet as a reward.

Ben—Weddings and funerals. (Seriously, both those occasions make me feel like I deserve to eat whatever I want!)

Karen—In the beginning, a stressful situation at work or at home would make me think "chocolate," but I wouldn't give in and now it really doesn't affect me anymore.

Joey—*Brady Bunch* reruns (I used to watch that show when I pigged out as a kid).

Dawn—Feeling tired or depressed.

Vicki—Social occasions. I love to eat when I'm entertaining, with friends, or when family is in town, and it's sometimes difficult when certain foods are around to tempt me and I'm not in my normal setting or keeping my regular schedule.

Emily—When I get sad, lonely, or down. (When I see this beginning I try to plan an outing or a day trip to the beach or mountains with my dogs. Fresh air and a little sunshine can work wonders.)

Jamie—Emotions.

Mark—Baseball games and the constant barrage of temptation. You know, "Peanuts, popcorn, nachos, cold beer here!"

Stephanie—Too much eating out.

Deb—Loneliness, anxiety, depression, and a need for comfort.

Margaret—Stress during PMS can cause them. However, for the most part, most of those old triggers and behaviors have faded away, or have become faint enough that they are much easier to deal with.

Paul—Sexual frustration.

Billi Jo—Emotional situations.

Ginger—Ice cream. I still have a sweet tooth at night. I have to fight the old "bad" habits wanting to creep back into my world. (When my mind tries to take over and tell my body it needs food to comfort it, my heart takes over and does the comforting.)

Larry—Nothing.

You Can Share Your Dreams

You can share your hopes and dreams with other people, but it's a good idea to be selective about who you share them with and how you share them. If you know that someone will probably react in a negative way, then you might be better off not telling them what you're planning. When it comes to people who are close to you, though, most of them will be happy for you, or at least want to be happy, but they might also be scared or nervous that your future won't include them or that they will not be as important to you as they are now.

Amy says, "When you make major changes in your own life, it always requires some rebalancing in your relationships. Whether those relationships are with friends, family members, or your partner, every relationship has a balance that partly has to do with how each person sees themselves and how they see each other.

"So, if you make a lot of changes, it can throw the people you're close to off balance, even if they're happy for you. Their best self might be celebrating for you, but at the same time they might be thinking, 'Oh my God, she's making so many changes. She's going to leave me in the dust. She's not going to love me anymore.' She's not going to want me to be their partner, friend, favorite sister, or whatever role they have. So you have to assume that although people will do their best to be happy for you, sometimes they may be unable to support further changes that you want to make. When you've lost weight, which is such a valuable piece of currency in the world, you're already stepping up and stepping out, so when you're getting ready to take other big steps in your life, it could easily make some of your loved ones nervous because they are afraid of being left behind."

In other words, if you're a two-year-old and you're learning to walk, your parents are going to cheer you on and be very excited about every step you take without falling. But they aren't necessarily going to be as purely happy when you move out of the house or go off to college, because you're leaving them and going on to bigger and better things and they're suddenly left with a big hole in their lives.

Thinking along those lines, Amy says, "If you want to elicit support for making further changes in your life, a smart thing to do is to include the people you care about as much as you can from the beginning. Tell them how important their support is to you and reassure them that you appreciated their past support and couldn't have made your past changes without them. Let them know how essential they are in your life. The key is to validate and reinforce their participation before you even start to take new steps toward your dream, so they feel less nervous about losing you from their lives. Once you reassure them about their importance in your life and your appreciation for their support in the past, tell them what your goals or dreams are for the future and ask them directly for the kind of support that you want. If you're the type of person who has trouble sticking with a plan, you might ask people to check in with you periodically about how you're doing. You can also ask people to celebrate with you when you take a significant step."

I used to have a dream, like a Cinderella story, of going away for a year and coming home thin. I actually got to live that to some degree and it did not work. I went away to a diet program out of town and came back a different person. I wasn't used to me and my friends weren't used to me. Some people even tried to sabotage me. It was only later, when I dieted at home and included my friends in my change, that it all worked out for the best. I had a chance to get used to my changes gradually and so did they. It felt safe and secure for all of us.

Amy says, "People *do* want to support each other's hopes and dreams, but it's important to remember that change makes people nervous, and if someone isn't able to give you the support you're seeking, it's usually their own insecurities that get in the way of being able to do it."

So if people are having a hard time giving you support, you shouldn't think that they don't love you or want you to make changes or progress. Amy explains, "They're probably just nervous that you're not going to love or need them anymore—it doesn't mean that they don't want good things for you. If that happens with several people who are part of your life, try to broaden the field of who you're seeking support from. Sometimes you need to find people who are less involved with you and whose lives will be less affected by the changes that you make." I call those people acquaintances. I love making new acquaintances and talking with people at Starbucks every day and having other light relationships. Acquaintances don't know how to press your buttons, so Starbucks is a safe and friendly atmosphere. Don't get me wrong, there is nothing like lifelong friends, but sometimes acquaintances have a lot of value for me.

Amy says, "Before you tell someone the details of your dreams, take them aside and tell them a little about what your goals are so you can gauge whether they will be able to support you. If you get a really negative reaction from someone, try to disconnect from that person with regard to that issue. People who have a negative attitude or initial response to your plans are not likely to be successfully engaged in an argument to the contrary, so there's rarely any point to trying to convince them or get them on board."

THE IMPERFECT TEN

The Top Ten Ways to Feed Your Dreams

1. Create a circle of support.
2. Don't dwell on the past or live in the future, but live the moments in between.
3. Don't compare yourself or your progress with others. (This was a major downfall of mine in the past.)
4. Clean up the wreckage of your past a little at a time by making amends with people and forgiving yourself and others.
5. Figure out exactly what your dreams are—the old and the new.
6. At the end of each day, ask yourself what one thing you can do to feed your dreams tomorrow.
7. Don't make excuses or say things to yourself like, "I should be here by now," or "It's too late." (As long as you're alive it's not too late! I know a heavy older woman who always tells me, "If only I were your age I could do it." That's bull. I could say the same thing to someone who is twenty years younger than I am.)
8. Have the same respect for yourself as others have for you!
9. Get stuffed on life! Get full from all the new projects you are working on, making your life more full of

> people, support, and new relationships. Now that's
> a good kind of full!
>
> **10.** The best way to feed your dreams is not to overfeed
> yourself. (It sounds simple, but you know it's not.)

Let's Stay in the Winners' Circle Forever!

One of the most simple but profound sayings I've ever
heard is, "Where there is a will, there is a way." One of the
best ways to strengthen your will and keep it strong is to figure out how maintaining your weight will help you to live
your hopes and dreams. There are very few things we can do
without our health, so that's a big one right there. Having
less weight to carry around also means you have more energy to put into your projects and the steps that will lead you
to the type of life you want to create for yourself. Hopes and
dreams have a magic all their own because they work two
ways for us. Having them keeps us motivated and gives our
life meaning, and maintaining our weight and our health
makes it easier and more fun for us to pursue and achieve
them.

Those of us in the Winners' Circle know that the potential for greatness really does live within us. Throughout this
book you've gotten to know a little about other people in
the Winners' Circle and what they are doing to keep winning. I'm hoping that you will be helped by their tips, and
also by knowing that you are part of a circle of winners. You

don't know each other personally, but you know a lot about each other's struggles and triumphs. (Those of us with food issues and addictions are very much alike.) We have many things in common and have experienced things—both bad and good—that a lot of people can't even begin to relate to or understand. During the times when you feel alone, you must learn to ask for people on your Winning Team to help you! I guarantee they will be there for you, but you have to form the words "I need help." And don't be ashamed; we all need help. (I think of Princess Diana a lot and how much she had to suffer with her eating problems alone.) It's true that the statistics for regaining weight are not in our favor, but it's also true that many people beat those odds, and we can beat them, too.

Remember that the two most important secrets to success are in our mind and in our heart. Where our mind and heart lead us, our body will follow. There are no exceptions to that rule. By practicing our game plan every day and refusing to give up, we will keep winning. To live our lives to the fullest, we need to stay strong, fit, and healthy. We have the will. We have the power. And we can stay in the Winners' Circle forever!

Won't you join me in the Winners' Circle? Please feel free to write me anytime at www.staceyhalprin.com. Your stories keep me going and it is my deepest wish that I have been some help to you.

Afterword

My home, the Big Apple, is known as the city that never sleeps, but I think they should call it the city that overeats! At 3 a.m. you can simply walk across the street and get steak on a stick, a hot pretzel, or a slice of pizza. It's a city where takeout menus are slipped under your door daily and restaurants deliver every type of food in the world all night long. The fact that I have been able to maintain my weight for five years while living in a twenty-four-hour smorgasbord makes me believe that everyone who really wants to win this battle, and is willing to do what it takes, can do it! That I was able to go from being nearly immobile to living a full, active life and writing my first book on maintaining weight loss makes me believe, beyond a shadow of a doubt, that all things are possible!

When I first began my weight loss journey, it was still very hard for me to get around, so my mother bought me two hook rug projects so I would have something to do and be able to make beautiful decorations for my apartment at the same time. (To be honest, I had no idea what to do with hands that only knew how to shovel food in my mouth over and over, so having something new to do with them made all the difference in the world.) The first project, a pillow with colorful flowers, I proudly finished and placed on my living room sofa. (It's still there today.) The second project, a wall hanging of a leopard, is still only about halfway done. At first I felt guilty for not finishing it, but then I realized that I didn't finish it because I had regained my mobility and was out living my life. I guess I felt it was more important to finish my life than to finish the wall hanging—and certainly life is more fun and interesting! I realized that not finishing it was actually a victory. Boy, was that an "Aha" moment! After all the years I spent alone and indoors, I treasure every single minute that I'm out in the world interacting with other people and experiencing everything life has to offer. I've discovered that I learned a lot more than I thought I did during my "hermit years," but now it's time for me to learn and grow with other people and to help other people to reclaim their lives by sharing what I've learned with them.

So many of the changes I've made in the past five years have nothing to do with food, but most of them have had an effect on the way I eat. I have become much more self-assured. I am outgoing and playful and have a good head on my shoulders. I hold my head high, start conversations with people, and I flirt—all qualities that come with a healthy sense of self.

But every so often something happens that really throws me for a loop and reminds me that I still have a way to go! One of those things was when my publisher said that they wanted to do a photo shoot and put my photo on the cover of this book. That shook my newfound confidence to the core. A lot of authors would jump for joy at that idea, but my world turned black. For some reason I felt like the fat lady all over again. Just the idea of my body being "on camera" and having all those people at a photo shoot focusing on my appearance made me shake.

On the day of the photo shoot, I tried to be calm, but my fears were lurking all around me. The shoot was in a stunning studio in the trendiest part of Manhattan. There was a full staff there, from photographers to lighting people and hair and makeup stylists, all to make my photo beautiful. I arrived with a suitcase full of clothing and jewelry as they asked me to do, but the people in charge of wardrobe said they had a different vision for the cover, so they sent one of their stylists out to find something simple but spectacular.

You see, since I had lost weight, I'd been dressing like somewhat of a sexpot. No one close to me had the guts or the heart to tell me my clothing choices were not the best; they were just happy I was healthy. I was anxious and curious to see what the stylist would return with, but when she walked in the door with a variety of white clothing, I thought I would die. I said, "Fat people can't wear white!" Everyone stopped and looked at me with confusion on their faces. Once again, I had gone back to thinking I was the fat lady, regardless of the reality of my current size.

Jeff, the makeup artist, who I had immediately bonded with at the beginning of the day, encouraged me to try on the outfits and promised he would be honest with me about how they looked. He also helped me to tone down the heavy makeup that no one except me felt I needed. He complimented me on each new outfit and the photographers and people on the set all smiled and told me that I honestly looked beautiful and it was the exact look they were going for. I felt very flattered when they explained that the look captured my personality—classy, sexy, and sophisticated all wrapped up into one.

Several people on the crew gently tried to tell me how well this new look suited me. I finally had my light bulb moment. I did not need to dress sexy to be sexy, and it was finally time to try a new look and less makeup.

The crew was very happy with the photos they were getting and invited me to see the images, but I said no because I was afraid it would ruin my day. I explained that I had lost so much weight that I still wasn't able to completely shake my old self-image. The photographer looked at me and said, "Maybe you will never lose that image." Her words went through me like a chill. And they made me wonder. Will we, the people who make it to the stage where we're maintaining our weight loss, ever shake the old image?

After lunch, I told the crew that I was ready to look at just one picture. When I saw the photo I could not believe this classy, sexy woman in white was really me. It was the most gorgeous picture I had ever seen of myself. I asked if they had retouched the picture and they smiled and said no.

I left the studio that day feeling as light as a feather and knowing that I was no longer the fat girl I once was. I felt excited about creating yet another new me—a fresher, classier me. I learned some very important lessons that day and had a lot to think about.

As we grow to be more comfortable with our new size and continue to make other changes in our lives that are physically, mentally, and spiritually healthy, we discover new things about ourselves and from time to time we feel a need to make some more changes on the outside to reflect what's going on with us on the inside.

I knew for sure that what I had once heard was really true: "Life isn't about finding yourself. Life is about creating yourself." So here I go again!

Resources

The following resources have been compiled to support your ongoing success with maintaining your weight loss. In addition to contact information for all of the experts who provided me with information and guidance, you will find books, videos and DVDs, organizations, and Web sites that have more information about fitness and general health, food and nutrition, and mental health. I've also listed my own Web site and contact information so you can stay in touch, schedule or find out about my personal appearances, let me know how you're doing, share your success stories, or join the Winners' Circle!

Stacey Halprin
www.StaceyHalprin.com
212-414-5188

Experts

Doug Caporrino
Results thru Research
www.resultsthruresearch.com
866-GETTFIT (438-8348)

Dr. Andrew Elkwood
Plastic Surgery Center
Shrewsbury, NJ
www.looknatural.com

Dr. Jane Greer
www.drjanegreer.com
E-mail: DrGreer111@aol.com

Dr. Bruce Hoffman
The Hoffman Centre for Integrative Medicine
www.hoffmancentre.com
E-mail: info@hoffmancentre.com

Dr. Denise Ariahna Nadler
Healing Integrations
Think Better, Feel Better, Be Better
www.healingintegrations.com
E-mail: info@healingintegrations.com

Dr. Amy Ojerholm
E-mail: doctoramyo@yahoo.com
(212) 479-0879

Fitness and Health

Books

Anderson, Bob. *Stretching.* 20th Anniversary Revised Edition. Bolinas, CA: Shelter Publications, 2000.

Ansari, Mark. *Yoga for Beginners.* New York: HarperCollins, 1999.

Clarke, Michaela. *Ashtanga Yoga for Beginners.* London: Gaia, 2006.

Dreyer, Danny. *ChiRunning: A Revolutionary Approach to Effortless, Injury-Free Running.* New York: Simon and Schuster, 2004.

——— *ChiWalking: The Five Mindful Steps for Lifelong Health and Energy.* New York: Simon and Schuster, 2006.

Friedman, Philip, and Gail Eisen. *The Pilates Method of Physical and Mental Conditioning.* New York: Studio, 2004.

Greene, Bob. *Bob Greene's Total Body Makeover: An Accelerated Program of Exercise and Nutrition for Maximum Results in Minimum Time.* New York: Simon and Schuster, 2005.

Isaacs, Greg. *10,000 Steps a Day to Your Optimal Weight: Walk Your Way to Better Health.* Los Angeles: Bonus Books, 2006.

Kahn, June, and Lawrence Biscontini. *Morning Cardio Workouts.* Champaign, IL: Human Kinetics, 2006.

Kelley, Sheila. *The S Factor: Strip Workouts for Every Woman.* New York: Workman, 2003.

Kowalchik, Claire. *The Complete Book of Running for Women: Everything You Need to Know about Training, Nutrition, Injury Prevention, Motivation, Racing and Much, Much More.* New York: Simon and Schuster, 1999.

Lewis, Carole. *Age-Defying Fitness: Making the Most of Your Body for the Rest of Your Life.* Atlanta: Peachtree, 2006.

Ni, Maoshing. *Tai Chi.* San Francisco: Chronicle, 2006.

Northrup, Christiane, MD. *Women's Bodies, Women's Wisdom: Creating Physical and Emotional Health and Healing.* New York: Bantam, 2006.

Null, Gary. *Get Healthy Now!: A Complete Guide to Prevention, Treatment, and Healthy Living.* New York: Seven Stories, 2006.

Pagano, Joan. *Strength Training for Women: Tone up, Burn Calories, Stay Strong.* New York: DK Publishing, 2004.

Thurmond, Michael. *12-Day Body Shaping Miracle: Change Your Shape, Transform Problem Areas, and Beat Fat for Good.* New York: Warner Wellness, 2007.

Verstegen, Mark. *Core Performance Essentials: Twenty-Five Exercises to Create a Lean, Powerful, Injury-Resistant Physique for Life.* New York: Rodale, 2005.

Villepigue, James, and Hugo Rivera. *The Body Sculpting Bible for Men.* New York: Hatherleigh, 2002.

DVDs and Videos

Fat Chance Belly Dance
www.fatchancebellydance.com
PO Box 460594
San Francisco, CA 94146
E-mail: fcbd@earthlink.net
(415) 431–4322

Carolena Nericcio is credited with developing American Tribal Style Belly Dance and founded Fat Chance Belly Dance in 1987. Fat Chance Belly Dance instructional programs include Tribal Basics Dance Fundamentals, Zils, Advanced Workshop, Cues and Transitions, and Improvisational. Fitness VHS or DVDs include *Fat Chance Belly Dance Woman Power Workout* with Karen Andes and *Tribal Fusion Yoga, Isolations and Drills: A Practice Companion* with Rachel Brice.

Gentle Fitness
www.gentlefitness.com
732 Lake Shore Drive
Rhinelander, WI 54501
(800) 566–7780

Their award-winning videotape comes with a helpful twenty-page book. Blends yoga, tai chi, and Feldenkrais movement awareness. $28.70 including postage.

The S Factor
www.sfactor.com
5225 Wilshire Blvd., #B
Los Angeles, CA 90036
(323) 965–9685

Sheila Kelley, wife, mother, and actress, is the founder of the S Factor Movement. The DVD (or VHS) *S Factor 1: The Beginning* teaches the liberating movement technique that combines yoga, dance, and the athleticism and sexual expression of stripping to teach you a whole new way to move and view your body. Once you learn the basics, you can work your way up to *S Factor 2: Pole Work 101* and *Advanced Pole Work*!

Winsor Pilates
www.winsorpilates.com
Studio: 8204 Melrose Ave.
Los Angeles, CA 90046
(800) 747–3503

Mari Winsor, professional dancer and teacher, began developing her innovative workout nearly twenty years ago and opened her first Pilates studio in 1990 in Los Angeles with techniques based on the groundbreaking workout introduced by Joseph H. Pilates in the 1920s. Her exercise programs include *20 Minute Circle Workout*, *Accelerated Fat Burning Workout*, *Abs Workout*, *Bun & Thigh Workout*, and *Upper Body Sculpting*.

Online Stores

Natural Journeys
www.naturaljourneys.com
A division of Goldhil Entertainment
5284 Adolfo Road
Camarillo, CA 93012
(800) 737–1825

Natural Journeys offers a wide variety of dance, fitness, and martial arts instructional videotapes and DVDs, including pregnancy fitness, back care, relaxation, and massage. Among the great selections is *Yoga for Beauty Dawn and Dusk* with Rainbeau Mars (2-DVD set). The *Dawn* DVD has fifty-eight moves for a strong, beautiful body! You'll learn energizing stretches to start the day and revitalize with powerful breathing techniques. The *Dusk* DVD teaches fifty-two ways to relax and relieve tension, cleansing poses to detoxify your body, and healing yoga and breathing exercises.

Collage Video
Exercise Video Specialists
www.collagevideo.com
5930 Main St. NE
Minneapolis, MN 55421
(800) 433–6769

Collage Video offers more than seven hundred videos and DVDs on a wide variety of fitness programs including aerobics, toning, step, Pilates, yoga, stretch, dance, kickboxing, ballet, and the stability ball. You can preview any video for 60 seconds for free and everything you order has a thirty-day satisfaction guarantee. Collage Video says, "We've physically *done* every one of these videos. That's how we know they're the best of the thousands of workouts we've seen since 1987."

Games

The Fitness Challenge, Inc.
www.fitnesschallenge.com
(877) 724-2553

The Fitness Challenge is an exercise program packaged in the form of a colorful and fun game. The object of the game is for two people of any age or fitness level to challenge each other to participate in and complete an eight-week exercise program. The Fitness Challenge Foundation is a nonprofit organization whose mission is to promote health and wellness, medical research, and family and child welfare.

Web Sites

Caloriesperhour.com
www.caloriesperhour.com

Caloriesperhour offers information on weight loss, metabolism, genetics, eating disorders, exercise, spot reducing, cellulite, and surgery. The site provides a calculator for calories burned by a wide variety of daily activities and exercises; a food calories and nutrition calculator that calculates calories, protein, fat, carbohydrates, fiber, and sodium for over 23,200 foods from grocery stores, fast-food chains, and restaurants; and a weight loss calculator that calculates the time and daily calorie loss required to reach your goal weight. This site also has diet and weight loss forums where you can post questions, get support, and give support to others.

The Fitness Jumpsite!
Your connection to a lifestyle of fitness, nutrition, and health
www.primusweb.com/fitnesspartner/

The Fitness Jumpsite provides information on nutrition, weight management, fitness equipment, and advice and ideas for getting and staying active, including how to increase your daily activity, getting motivated, and turning up the intensity. It also provides specific workouts, a fitness library, and an Activity Calorie Calculator that includes sport and training activities as well as occupational and daily life activities.

Food and Nutrition

Books

Alexander, Devin. *The Biggest Loser Cookbook: More Than 125 Healthy, Delicious Recipes Adapted from NBC's Hit Show.* New York: Rodale, 2006.

Allport, Susan. *The Queen of Fats: Why Omega-3s Were Removed from the Western Diet and What We Can Do to Replace Them.* Berkeley: University of California Press, 2006.

Balch, Phyllis A. *Prescription for Nutritional Healing.* New York: Penguin, 2006.

Davis, W. Marvin. *Consumer's Guide to Dietary Supplements and Alternative Medicines: Servings of Hope.* Binghamton, NY: Haworth, 2006.

Hobbs, Suzanne Havala. *Get the Trans Fat Out: 601 Simple Ways to Cut the Trans Fat Out of Any Diet.* New York: Three Rivers, 2006.

Kenney, Matthew, and Sarma Melngailis. *Raw Food/ Real World: 100 Recipes to Get the Glow.* New York: HarperCollins, 2005.

Kimbrell, Andrew. *Your Right to Know: Genetic Engineering and the Secret Changes in Your Food.* San Rafael, CA: Mandala, 2006.

Lieberman, Shari. *The Gluten Connection: How Gluten Sensitivity May Be Sabotaging Your Weight and Your Health—And What You Can Do to Take Control Now.* New York: Rodale, Press 2006.

McGraw, Phillip C. *The Ultimate Weight Solution Food Guide.* New York: Simon and Schuster, 2003.

Murray, Michael, Joseph E. Pizzorno, and Lara U. Pizzorno. *The Encyclopaedia of Healing Foods.* New York: Simon and Schuster, 2006.

Somer, Elizabeth. *Nutrition for a Healthy Pregnancy: The Complete Guide to Eating Before, During, and After Your Pregnancy.* Revised Edition. New York: Henry Holt, 2002.

Steinman, David. *Diet for a Poisoned Planet: How to Choose Safe Foods for You and Your Family.* New York: Thunder's Mouth, 2006.

Tessmar, Kimberly. *No-Sugar Cookbook: Delicious Recipes to Make Your Mouth Water . . . All Sugar Free.* Avon, MA: Adams Media Corporation, 2006.

Weil, Andrew, MD. *Eating Well for Optimum Health: The Essential Guide to Bringing Health and Pleasure Back to Eating.* New York: HarperCollins, 2001.

Weil, Andrew, MD, and Rosie Daley. *The Healthy Kitchen: Recipes for a Better Body, Life, and Spirit.* New York: Knopf, 2002.

Young, Robert O., and Shelley Redford Young. *The pH Miracle for Weight Loss: Balance Your Body Chemistry, Achieve Your Ideal Weight.* New York: Warner Books, 2005.

Web Sites

Calories Information
www.calorie-counter.net

Provides information about nutrition and calories in food, calorie needs to maintain or lose weight, how many calories are burned by exercise and fitness equipment, advice about which exercise is best for weight loss, guidelines on calorie intake for children and teens, and information on how much exercise is needed to burn off certain foods.

Consumers Union
Nonprofit publisher of *Consumer Reports*
www.consumersunion.org

Provides information on food contaminants, genetically engineered food, mad cow disease, organic food, pesticides and integrated pest management, and food labeling. Consumers Union states that "Consumers Union's food safety efforts seek to focus public attention on food safety risks and regulatory deficiencies that can result in harm to the public. You can take action on food safety by visiting our sister site, www.notinmyfood.org."

My Pyramid
www.mypyramid.gov

The My Pyramid site can help you choose the foods and amounts that are right for you. Get a quick estimate of what and how much you need to eat, based on information you enter for age, sex, and activity level. This site is owned and operated by the Center for Nutrition Policy and Promotion, an organization of the U.S. Department of Agriculture. It was established to improve the nutrition and well-being of Americans. The center's two primary objectives are to advance and promote dietary guidance and to conduct applied research and analyses in nutrition and consumer economics.

Nature's First Law Online Superstore
www.rawfood.com

This Web site sells and offers information about organic, wild foods, and/or superfoods in their raw natural state. Nature's First Law states that "eating a balanced mix of raw plant foods restores the body on a molecular level, building strong cells, radically naturalizing the body, raising alkalinity, and grounding the person in the natural world."

Zone Chefs
www.zonechefs.com
(800) 939-0663
Zone Chefs will deliver delicious healthy food to your door.

Mental Health

Books

BenShea, Noah. *A COMPASS for Healing: Finding Your Way from Emotional Pain to Peace.* New York: Health Communications, 2006.

Braverman, Eric R. *Younger You: Unlock the Hidden Power of Your Brain to Look and Feel 15 Years Younger.* New York: McGraw-Hill, 2006.

Danowski, Debbie. *When Enough Is Enough: 90 Truths You Need to Stop Emotional Eating and Start Living Well.* New York: Avalon, 2006.

Demartini, John F. *Heart of Love: How to Go Beyond Fantasy to Find True Relationship Fulfillment.* Carlsbad, CA: Hay House, 2006.

Hartman, Thom. *Walking Your Blues Away: Practical Bilateral Therapies for Healing the Mind and Optimizing Emotional Well-Being.* Rochester, VT: Inner Traditions International, 2006.

Hemingway, Mariel. *Healthy Living from the Inside Out: Every Woman's Guide to Real Beauty, Renewed Energy, and a Radiant Life.* New York: HarperCollins, 2006.

Honos-Webb, Lara. *Gift of Depression: How Listening to Your Pain Can Heal Your Life.* Oakland, CA: New Harbinger, 2006.

Janov, Arthur. *Primal Healing: Access the Incredible Power of Feelings to Improve Your Health.* Franklin Lakes, NJ: Career Press, 2006.

Katie, Byron, with Stephen Mitchell. *Loving What Is: Four Questions That Can Change Your Life.* New York: Crown, 2003.

Myss, Caroline. *Invisible Acts of Power: Channeling Grace in Your Everyday Life.* New York: Free Press, 2005.

Neeld, Elizabeth Harper. *Tough Transitions: Navigating Your Way Through Difficult Times.* New York: Warner Books, 2006.

Ruiz, Miguel. *The Four Agreements: A Practical Guide to Personal Freedom.* San Rafael, CA: Amber-Allen, 1997.

Schachter, Michael B. *What Your Doctor May Not Tell You About Depression: The Breakthrough All-Natural Solution for Effective Treatment.* New York: Warner Books, 2006.

Wasserman, Danuta. *Depression: The Facts.* Oxford, England: Oxford University Press, 2006.

Weight Maintenance Web Sites and Online Forums

The National Weight Control Registry
www.nwcr.ws/

The National Weight Control Registry is a U.S. register of people (eighteen years or older) who have lost at least 14 kilograms (30 pounds) of weight and kept it off for at least one year. This site also includes research reports and the opportunity to participate in a variety of studies.

CureZone
www.curezone.org

This Web site offers links to hundreds of support and health forums, including:

Dr. Phil McGraw: The Ultimate Weight Solution:
  The 7 Keys to Weight Loss Freedom
Weight Reduction—Weight Control Forum
The Zone Diet Support—Barry Sears
Exercise and Fitness Support Forum
Bariatric Surgery/Gastric Bypass Forum—Weight Loss
  Surgery Resources
Raw Food for Weight Loss Support Forum

Other Forums Worth Checking Out

3 Fat Chicks on a Diet Weight Loss Community
www.3fatchicks.com/forum
(This Web site also has a chat room.)

Caloriesperhour.com
www.caloriesperhour.com

DietPower Forums
"Share Ideas, Make Friends"
www.forums.dietpower.com

Healthy Weight Forum
www.healthyweightforum.org

To Lobby for Changes in Insurance Coverage

If you believe that insurance companies should cover the costs of reconstructive surgeries following significant amounts of weight loss, let your representatives know how you feel by writing them a letter!

FirstGov.gov
The U.S. government's official Web portal
www.firstgov.gov

This Web site provides information for how to contact the president and vice president of the United States and how to find out who your state governor, senators, representatives, and legislators are and obtain their contact information.

Index

addictions
    hoarding behavior, 242–43
    recovery and living in "day-tight"
        compartments, 196
    replacing eating with another
        addiction, 91–93
affirmations, 71
    changing negative self-talk and
        thoughts, 199–200
    "today is a new day," 196
Aristotle, 155

Bach, Richard, xvii
Big D's (Decisions, Deadlines,
    Disappointments, Disasters),
    179–83
binge eating
    crisis triggering, limiting the
        damage, 160–61
    denial and triggering, 152
    exercise and, 161
    knowing your overeating triggers,
        248–50
    responding to, 192
    stress and, 21
    using as a delay tactic, 159–60
body image, 113–16, 260–61
    desensitization exercise, 114–16
    plastic surgery and, 117–19
    shame and, 149
breathing exercise (Nadi Shodhana),
    24–25

calories
    bagel substitution, 162
cake substitution, 162
cheese substitution, 163
chocolate substitution, 163–64
cookie substitution, 164
doughnut substitution, 165
exercise needed to burn daily
    intake, 52–53
fats, maximum per day, 45
frappuccino with whipped cream
    substitution, 165
ice cream substitution, 165
Jody's daily decrease of calories to
    counteract weight gain, 167–68
Newman's Own low-fat cookies
    and fat-free Fig Newtons,
    162–66
piece of candy substitution,
    162–63
pie substitution, 166
regular yogurt substitution, 167
snack bag of potato chips
    substitution, 166
soda substitution, 166
substitutions for temptations,
    162–68
Web site calculators, 52, 53, 54
Caporrino, Doug, xxxii
    fitness plan, 56–67
    food choices, 46–47
    lactic acid build-up, tips for
        reducing, 51
    stretching guidelines, 65–66
clothes and makeup, 214–23
    avoiding fashion faux pas,
        216–17, 259–60

clothes and makeup (*continued*)
  black vs. color, 218–21
  choosing makeup, 223, 260
  digital photos for a new look, 215
  downsizing wardrobe, 220–21
  five-year-rule, 221–22
  free department store makeovers,
    222
  hairstyle, 221–22
  personal shoppers, 215
  variety vs. trends, 217–18
cortisol: stress and, 19–21

daily program (one day at a time),
    193–225
  discover the beauty of your flaws,
    201, 203–5
  keeping your love life fresh,
    213–14
  living in "day-tight"
    compartments, 196
  living in the moment, 210–11
  paper trail to better health, 205–9
  red flags of weight gain, 212
  start fresh, finish strong, 195–200
  staying open to possibilities, 205,
    209–11
  style sense, defining and refining,
    214–23
  Top Ten Ways to Start Your Day
    Fresh and Finish Strong,
    222–25
depression: obesity and, xxiv
Descartes, Rene, 83
Diana, Princess of Wales, 256
dreams (goals), 226–56
  changing, 231–33
  changing, effect on relationships,
    251–53
  dreams reached by Winners' Circle
    members, 229–30
  feeding, to feel full, 228–33
  helping others, 229, 241–45
  identifying, 232, 235–39

leap of faith and, 227
love relationship, identifying and
    finding, 227, 245–48
purpose statement, 238–39
pursuing, 234–35
reaching beyond yourself,
    240–45
sharing with others, 250–53
three action steps, 239
Top Ten Ways to Feed Your
    Dreams, 254–55
Dress Code, The (film), 194

eating out
  asking for take-home box at start
    of meal, 99–100
  tips for, 20
Elkwood, Andrew, xxxii–xxxiii,
    117–19, 205–9
emotions
  accepting the things you cannot
    change, 100–103
  accepting weight loss, 11
  anger at past rejection, 11–12
  attributing your problems to
    being overweight, 94
  bag of tricks for, 171–74
  being proactive about your needs,
    111
  Big D's (Decisions, Deadlines,
    Disappointments, Disasters),
    179–83
  body image and, 113–16
  celebrating victories, building
    emotional strength with,
    130–38
  common issues on "Learn to
    Accept" lists, 102–3
  coping with regrets, 97–98
  distracting yourself from negative
    emotions, 98–99
  a dozen paths to empowerment,
    108–13
  exercise as means to change, 160

FEAR (False Emotions Appearing Real), 135
food and, xxv, xxvii, 157–58, 181–82, 212
introducing family and friends to the new you, 88–90
journaling and, 14–16
living in the moment, 31, 210–11
mind-body connection, 36
"negative forecasting," 209–11
negativity and stress, 134–35
overeating and, 84–85, 96, 248–50
psychotherapy for issues, 87
replacing eating with another addiction and, 91–93
sexuality and, 120–24
stress and, 18–19
Three-Day Time-Out and, 183–88
Top Ten Reasons to Turn Your Pain into Power, 123–24
turning pain into power, 83–124
using affirmations to change feelings, 199–200
validating feelings, 180
verbalizing feelings instead of swallowing, 13–14, 16
See also relationships
empowerment, a dozen paths to, 108–13
exercise and physical fitness
breathing exercise (Nadi Shodhana), 24–25, 24n
calculating daily requirements, 52–53, 146
cardiovascular training, 57–60
to change emotional state, 160
choosing most enjoyable, 50–51
to counteract bingeing, 161
daily, incorporating, 67–68
flexibility training, 51, 65–67
"good tired," 52
heart rate, how to determine, 57–58

Internet calories-burned calculators, 52, 53, 54
lactic acid build-up, tips for reducing, 51
lowering stress level with, 24
maintenance plan, 49–67
Margaret's daily routine, 229
"no pain, no gain," 51
Optimum Fitness List, 79–80
options to choose from, 53–57
pedometer for, 70
physical injury, dealing with, 169–71
post-session activities to prevent soreness, 51
stepping up your plan, 202–3
strength training, 60–65
stretching guidelines, 65–66
swimming, 59–60
walking, jogging, or cycling, 58–59

Fitness Challenge game, 53–57

gastric bypass surgery, xxii–xxiii
goals. See dreams (goals)
goal weight
adjusting, 37–38
Internet resources for healthiest weight range, 39
stepping up your plan and, 202
ways maintaining goal weight is beneficial list, 237–39
Greer, Jane, xxxi–xxxii
"before and after" exercise, 7–8
creating sexual connections, 121–23
dream mate, 246–48
feeding your heart and soul, 26–27
keeping your love life fresh, 213–14
rebounding from rejection, 175–78
writing your own script, 70–72

Hoffman, Bruce, xxxiii
Hoffman Centre for Integrative
    Medicine, Calgary, xxxiii
Hughes, Langston, 226

*Illusions: The Adventures of a Reluctant
    Messiah* (Bach), xvii
insulin: stress and, 19–22
Internet resources
    calories-burned calculators, 52–53
    for healthiest weight range, 39
    online discussion groups, 6
    USDA mypyramid.gov Web site, 46
    Winners' Circle, 255

James, William, 36
Jenny Craig Weight Loss Program,
    152–53
    commercials, Winners' Circle
        women in, 152, 230
journaling, 14–16
    as delay strategy, 15
    emotions, 14
    validating yourself in, 16
    See also Winners' Circle Workbook

Kafka, Franz, 125

La Lanne, Jack, 46
laughter, 37
    empowerment and, 109–10
lifestyle changes
    balancing improvement with
        acceptance, 68–70
    being real with yourself and,
        144–46
    daily exercise, 67–68
    Do List, 71
    exercise maintenance plan, 49–67
    living in the moment, 31
    nutrition for life, 39–41
    plan enjoyable activities, 27–30,
        36–37
    proactive approach, 70–72

stepping up your plan, 203
style sense, defining and refining,
    214–23
Top Ten Worst Reasons for Not
    Making a Winning Game Plan,
    80–82
Lombardi, Vince, 32

maintenance plan, 32–82
    avoiding excuses for eating, 31
    avoiding starving, 31
    balancing improvement with
        acceptance, 68–70
    exercise, 34, 49–67
    Game Plan Assessment, 38
    knowing your overeating triggers,
        248–50
    list of excuses, 73–75
    low-fat or no-fat food
        substitutions, 162–68
    mental challenge, believing you
        can succeed, 35–38
    mental health, 34
    monitoring your weight, 75–76
    nutrition and diet, 34, 39–49
    pre-planning eating out, 20, 30
    regrouping after gaining a few
        pounds, 96–97
    shopping when not hungry, 31
    sticking to planning for, 30
    tips from the Winners' Circle, 77
    Top Ten Worst Reasons for Not
        Making a Winning Game Plan,
        80–82
    weighing yourself, 31, 75–76, 144,
        167
    writing out your plan, 78–80
    writing your own script, 70–72
maintenance plan, dealing with
        challenges and set-backs,
        155–92
    before and after pictures,
        174–75
    bag of tricks for, 171–74

Big D's (Decisions, Deadlines, Disappointments, Disasters), 179–83
binge eating, 159–61
dealing with a curveball: using your senses, 157–61
delay tactics for temptation, 159–60
getting help when needed, 191
marital status change, 168–69
motivation, 175, 228–33, 237–39
physical injury, 169–71
rebounding from rejection, 175–78
smart alternatives for food choices, 161–66
Three-Day Time-Out, 183–88
Top Ten Tips to Stay in the Game, 192
water healing transformation process, 188–91
weight gain, immediate response, 167–68
mental health, 34
bag of tricks for, 171–74
believing you can succeed, 35–38
menu, creating (Do List), 72
plan enjoyable activities, 27–30, 36–37
mind-body relationship, 35–36
Molecules of Emotion (Pert), 36
motivation, 175, 228–33, 237–39

Nadler, Denise Ariahna, xxxii
on being your own champion, 148–49
on body language, 147
empowerment, paths to, 108–10
getting in touch with your dreams, 235, 236–39
on mind-body connection, 35–36, 72
water healing transformation process, 188–91

nutrition and diet, 39–49
boundaries for eating habits, 140–42
carbohydrates, 41–42
carbohydrates, best sources, 42
carbohydrates, percent of diet, 41–42
dairy foods, 47
diet soda, 47
fats, 45–46
fats, maximum calories per day, 45
favorite foods, rewarding yourself with, 170
fish warning, 45
low-fat food, 34, 40
low-fat or no-fat food substitutions, 162–68
omega-3 fatty acids, 45
Optimum Nutrition List, 78–79
organic foods, 44, 46–47
proteins, 42–44
proteins, complementary vs. complete, 43
proteins, non-meat sources, 44
proteins, percent of diet, 43
raw foods, 46
slips from, dealing with, 31, 77, 135, 140
snack size versus full size purchases, 170
Stacey's Top Ten Foods Banned from the House, 48–49
tips from the Winners' Circle, 77
tips to avoid temptation, 47–49
USDA guidelines, 40–41
USDA mypyramid.gov Web site, 46
water, 41, 47, 136–37

OA (Overeaters Anonymous), 95, 97
Ojerholm, Amy, xxvii, xxxi
attributing your problems to being overweight, 94

Ojerholm, Amy (*continued*)
  balancing improvement with
    acceptance, 68–70
  bingeing during a crisis, 160–61
  on body image, 113–14
  changing goals, effect on
    relationships, 251–53
  dealing with a curveball: using
    your senses, 157–58
  dealing with the Big D's, 180
  desensitization exercise, 114–16
  empowerment, paths to, 110–12
  experiencing emotional loss,
    105–6
  finding support, 16
  finding your authentic voice, 14
  first year difficulties, 130, 132
  giving yourself credit and self-
    esteem, 135–36
  "negative forecasting," 209–11
Old You and the New You, 3–6
  acknowledge your support team, 6
  "before and after" exercise, 7–8
  dental care and, 28
  introducing family and friends to
    the new you, 88–90
  listing what you feel proud of, 4–6
  love affair with the world and,
    25–28
  planning feel-good activities,
    27–30
  relationships, changing, 9–18
  shedding the invisibility cloak,
    9–13
  stopping stress, 18–25
Oprah, xxiv, 36

patience, 136–38
Pert, Candace P., 36
plastic or reconstructive surgery, 103
  choosing a surgeon, 118–19
  excess skin and, 117–19, 205–9
  preparing for, 210
positive attitude, 126, 130–38

changing negative self-talk and
    thoughts, 199–200
  helping others and, 241–45
Proust, Marcel, 1
psychotherapy
  emotional issues and, 87
  empowering yourself and, 112
Pure Food and Wine restaurant, 46

relationships
  attractiveness to partners, 86
  boundaries, establishing, 18
  changing goals, effect on
    relationships, 251–53
  dating and meeting new people,
    86–87
  ending, 103–6
  former "eating buddies," 9,
    12–13, 103–4
  "good enemy," 108
  introducing family and friends to
    the new you, 88–90
  jealousy of siblings and friends, 9
  leaving the past and, 17
  love partners, 213–14, 227, 245–48
  partners feeling threatened by
    your weight loss, 9, 10
  people pleasing, 243–44
  renewing good ones and re-
    creating others, 106–8
  self-confidence and body
    language, 146–49, 153
  unsolicited feedback, dealing
    with, 17–18
  weight loss and parents, 85–86
  weight loss sabotaged by, 9–13
Rochefoucauld, François Duc de la,
    193

self-esteem
  acting confident as strategy,
    148–49
  body image and, 113–19
  challenges to, 258–59

clothes, makeup and, 223
a dozen paths to empowerment,
    108–13
eating attitudes and, 30–31
giving yourself credit and, 135–36
growing in comfort, confidence,
    and self-respect, 146–49
helping others and, 229
planning feel-good activities,
    27–30
practicing patience with yourself,
    136–38
sexuality and, 116
stress and tendency to be negative,
    134–35
Top Ten Small Victories Worth
    Celebrating, 153–54
sexuality
    body image and, 115–16
    creating sexual connections,
        121–23
    sexual roadblocks and dating dead
        ends, 175
    increasing satisfaction, 120–21
    keeping your love life fresh,
        213–14
    rebounding from rejection,
        175–78
skin care, 142–44
sneak eating, 139
Sorensen, Vicki, 53–54
"So What?" syndrome, 241
stress
    action plan for stress-free eating,
        22–24
    binge eating and, 21
    breathing exercise for, 24–25
    checking on emotions and, 18–19
    cortisol, insulin, and weight gain,
        19–22
    exercise to lower, 24–25
    laughter to reduce, 37
    negativity and, 134–35
    overeating and, 19

support groups/individuals
    articulating your issues with, 17
    getting help when needed, 30, 191
    ongoing struggles and, 16–17
    online discussion groups, 6
    "phone a friend" lifeline, 148
    problems that don't disappear
        with the pounds and, 94–95
    sharing your dreams, 250–53

Tannen, Florence, 95–97
teeth: caring for, 28
Three-Day Time-Out, 183–88
thyroid function: stress, weight gain,
    and, 21
tyrosine, 21

victories, celebrating, 125–54
    accomplishments from the
        Winners' Circle, 139–42
    being real with yourself and,
        144–46
    building emotional strength with,
        130–38
    documenting and sharing,
        126–28
    enjoying what you used to dread,
        129–30
    Ginger's story, 152–53
    growing in comfort, confidence,
        and self-respect, 146–49
    identifying your
        accomplishments, 138–39
    sample list, 128
    taking joy in simple pleasures,
        150–51
    Top Ten Small Victories Worth
        Celebrating, 153–54

water, 41, 47
    tip for making it easier, 136–37
    using as a delay tactic, 159
water healing transformation
    process, 188–91

weighing yourself, 31, 75–76, 144, 167

weight gain
changing habits and, 146
daily calorie decreasing for weight gain, 167–68
exercise increase daily, 167
facing with honesty, 144–46
immediate response, 167–68
red flags, 212
regrouping after gaining a few pounds, 96–97
substitutions for temptations, 162–68

Weight Loss Surgery Support Group, St. Luke's-Roosevelt Hospital Center, xxxi

Winners' Circle, xxix
accomplishments to celebrate, 139–42
downsizing your wardrobe advice, 220–21
dreams reached by members, 229–30
enjoying what they used to dread, 129–30
exercise as part of daily life, 50, 54
feeling "more like themselves," 147
joining, 254–55
lifestyle changes, 34
list of simple pleasures, 151
lost friendships after weight loss, 104–5
overeating triggers of, 248–50
paying attention to the good things, 131–32
practicing moderation, 144
random acts of kindness by, 245
red flags of weight gain, 212

relationships after weight loss, 86
sexual roadblocks and dating dead ends, 175
shedding the invisibility cloak, 9–13
tips for weight maintenance, 77
Top Ten Things Winners' Circle People Have In Common, 30–31
Web site, 255

Winners' Circle Workbook
accomplishments list, 138–39
change/acceptance list, 100–101
daily list: things to be grateful for, 198
do list, 72
dream relationship, describing, 247–48
exercise progress, 80
foods banned from the house, 48
game plan assessment, 38
"Hopes and Dreams" section, 235–39
list of excuses, 73–75
maintaining goal weight is beneficial list, 237–39
maintenance plan, 78–80
promise to stay in the game, 157
purpose statement, 238–39
simple pleasures list, 151
small victories recorded, 127–28
"Things I Want to Change/Improve" list, 100, 101, 200
"Things I Want to Learn to Accept" list, 100–101, 102–3
three action steps toward your dreams, 239
what you feel proud of list, 4–6
"Ya, buts" list, 198, 200